Study of Microbiological Safety in the Food Chain

Study of Microbiological Safety in the Food Chain

Editor

Nevijo Zdolec

MDPI • Basel • Beijing • Wuhan • Barcelona • Belgrade • Manchester • Tokyo • Cluj • Tianjin

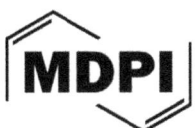

Editor
Nevijo Zdolec
University of Zagreb
Croatia

Editorial Office
MDPI
St. Alban-Anlage 66
4052 Basel, Switzerland

This is a reprint of articles from the Special Issue published online in the open access journal *Processes* (ISSN 2227-9717) (available at: https://www.mdpi.com/journal/processes/special_issues/Microbiological_Food).

For citation purposes, cite each article independently as indicated on the article page online and as indicated below:

LastName, A.A.; LastName, B.B.; LastName, C.C. Article Title. *Journal Name* **Year**, *Volume Number*, Page Range.

ISBN 978-3-0365-3070-3 (Hbk)
ISBN 978-3-0365-3071-0 (PDF)

Cover image courtesy of Nevijo Zdolec.

© 2022 by the authors. Articles in this book are Open Access and distributed under the Creative Commons Attribution (CC BY) license, which allows users to download, copy and build upon published articles, as long as the author and publisher are properly credited, which ensures maximum dissemination and a wider impact of our publications.

The book as a whole is distributed by MDPI under the terms and conditions of the Creative Commons license CC BY-NC-ND.

Contents

About the Editor vii

Preface to "Study of Microbiological Safety in the Food Chain" ix

Nevijo Zdolec
Introduction to Special Issue: Study of Microbiological Safety in the Food Chain
Reprinted from: *Processes* **2022**, *10*, 149, doi:10.3390/pr10010149 1

Nevijo Zdolec and Marta Kiš
Meat Safety from Farm to Slaughter—Risk-Based Control of *Yersinia enterocolitica* and *Toxoplasma gondii*
Reprinted from: *Processes* **2021**, *9*, 815, doi:10.3390/pr9050815 5

Sejeong Kim, Jong-Chan Kim, Sunhyun Park, Jinkwi Kim, Yohan Yoon and Heeyoung Lee
Identification of Microbial Flora in Dry Aged Beef to Evaluate the Rancidity during Dry Aging
Reprinted from: *Processes* **2021**, *9*, 2049, doi:10.3390/pr9112049 19

Tina Lešić, Nada Vahčić, Ivica Kos, Manuela Zadravec, Dragan Milićević, Irena Perković, Eddy Listeš and Jelka Pleadin
The Influence of Surface Mycobiota on Sensory Properties of "Istarski pršut" and "Dalmatinski pršut"
Reprinted from: *Processes* **2021**, *9*, 2287, doi:10.3390/pr9122287 27

Jana Výrostková, Ivana Regecová, Mariana Kováčová, Slavomír Marcinčák, Eva Dudriková and Jana Maľová
Antimicrobial Resistance of *Lactobacillus johnsonii* and *Lactobacillus zeae* in Raw Milk
Reprinted from: *Processes* **2020**, *8*, 1627, doi:10.3390/pr8121627 43

Andrea Lauková, Valentína Focková and Monika Pogány Simonová
Enterococcal Species Associated with Slovak Raw Goat Milk, Their Safety and Susceptibility to Lantibiotics and Durancin ED26E/7
Reprinted from: *Processes* **2021**, *9*, 681, doi:10.3390/pr9040681 57

Nevijo Zdolec, Tanja Bogdanović, Krešimir Severin, Vesna Dobranić, Snježana Kazazić, Jozo Grbavac, Jelka Pleadin, Sandra Petričević and Marta Kiš
Biogenic Amine Content in Retailed Cheese Varieties Produced with Commercial Bacterial or Mold Cultures
Reprinted from: *Processes* **2022**, *10*, 10, doi:10.3390/pr10010010 67

Andrea Lauková, Lenka Micenková, Monika Pogány Simonová, Valentína Focková, Jana Ščerbová, Martin Tomáška, Emília Dvorožňáková and Miroslav Kološta
Microbiome Associated with Slovak Traditional Ewe's Milk Lump Cheese
Reprinted from: *Processes* **2021**, *9*, 1603, doi:10.3390/pr9091603 77

Soňa Demjanová, Pavlina Jevinová, Monika Pipová and Ivana Regecová
Identification of *Penicillium verrucosum*, *Penicillium commune*, and *Penicillium crustosum* Isolated from Chicken Eggs
Reprinted from: *Processes* **2021**, *9*, 53, doi:10.3390/pr9010053 85

Pavlina Jevinová, Monika Pipová, Ivana Regecová, Soňa Demjanová, Boris Semjon, Slavomír Marcinčák, Jozef Nagy and Ivona Kožárová
Effect of *Cladosporium cladosporioides* on the Composition of Mycoflora and the Quality Parameters of Table Eggs during Storage
Reprinted from: *Processes* **2021**, *9*, 613, doi:10.3390/pr9040613 . . . . **99**

Qiao Hu, Yuwen Fang, Jiajia Zhu, Wenjiao Xu and Kui Zhu
Characterization of *Bacillus* Species from Market Foods in Beijing, China
Reprinted from: *Processes* **2021**, *9*, 866, doi:10.3390/pr9050866 . . . . **117**

About the Editor

Nevijo Zdolec graduated from the Faculty of Veterinary Medicine at the University of Zagreb in 2002 and received his PhD in Food Science in 2007. He is currently an associate professor at the Faculty of Veterinary Medicine, University of Zagreb, teaching food hygiene and technology. He has published more than 100 scientific papers and book chapters, 60 of which are indexed in the Web of Science Core Collection/Scopus database. He served as the editor of the international book Fermented Meat Products: Health Aspects and guest editor of two special issues of the journals Biomed Research International and Processes. Dr. Zdolec is a member of the Editorial Board of the journal Processes. Dr. Zdolec has been an invited speaker and member of the scientific and organisational advisory boards of several international conferences. He has been involved in two international projects and several national projects. Currently, he is involved in two COST actions and three projects financed by the European funds. His research and professional interests are in meat inspection, foodborne pathogens, lactic acid bacteria, antimicrobial resistance and antimicrobial technologies.

Preface to "Study of Microbiological Safety in the Food Chain"

Ensuring microbiological safety in the food (of animal origin) chain is a challenging task due to the complex interactions among animals, humans and the environment. However, technological and analytical advances in recent years have provided a broader insight into microbiological hazards in the food chain and risk assessment. This book, based on the Special Issue "Study of Microbiological Safety in the Food Chain", presents scientific papers addressing microbiological hazards in the food chain, such as bacterial antimicrobial resistance, bacterial or fungal spoilage of foods, the antimicrobial potential of the indigenous microbiota, the aminogenic or amine-reducing capacity of the microbiota, and papers that apply novel methods to study the food microbiome or risk-based methods in pathogen control. Four papers focused on the microbiological aspects of milk and dairy products, three on meat and meat products, two on eggs, and one on various *market* foods. The *microorganisms* of interest were species of lactobacilli, enterococci and molds, Yersinia enterocolitica, Bacillus cereus and the general microbiota in certain foods. As Guest Editor, I hope that this book will provide relevant new insights to scientists and professionals working in the field of food microbiology and public health.

Nevijo Zdolec
Editor

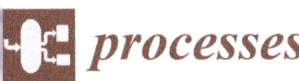

Editorial

Introduction to Special Issue: Study of Microbiological Safety in the Food Chain

Nevijo Zdolec

Department of Hygiene, Technology and Food Safety, Faculty of Veterinary Medicine, University of Zagreb, 10 000 Zagreb, Croatia; nzdolec@vef.hr; Tel.: +385-1-2390-193

Citation: Zdolec, N. Introduction to Special Issue: Study of Microbiological Safety in the Food Chain. *Processes* **2022**, *10*, 149. https://doi.org/10.3390/pr10010149

Received: 3 January 2022
Accepted: 11 January 2022
Published: 12 January 2022

Publisher's Note: MDPI stays neutral with regard to jurisdictional claims in published maps and institutional affiliations.

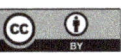

Copyright: © 2022 by the author. Licensee MDPI, Basel, Switzerland. This article is an open access article distributed under the terms and conditions of the Creative Commons Attribution (CC BY) license (https://creativecommons.org/licenses/by/4.0/).

Ensuring microbiological safety in the food (of animal origin) chain is a challenging task due to the complex interactions among animals, humans and the environment. However, technological and analytical advances in recent years have provided a broader insight into microbiological hazards in the food chain and risk assessment. The objective of the proposed Special Issue "Study of Microbiological Safety in the Food Chain" was therefore to obtain scientific papers addressing microbiological hazards in the food chain, such as bacterial antimicrobial resistance, bacterial or fungal spoilage of foods, the antimicrobial potential of the indigenous microbiota, and the aminogenic or amine-reducing capacity of the microbiota, and papers that apply novel methods to study the food microbiome to discover potential, previously unknown microbial hazards. The Special Issue of the journal Processes entitled "Study of Microbiological Safety in the Food Chain" consists of nine research papers and one review paper. Four papers focus on microbiological aspects of milk and dairy products, three on meat and meat products, two on eggs and one on various market foods. The microorganisms of interest were species of lactobacilli, enterococci and molds, *Yersinia enterocolitica*, *Bacillus cereus* and the general microbiota in certain foods.

Antimicrobial resistance has been one of the most important public health problems in recent years, and its transmission through the food chain is being investigated in many studies. In addition to foodborne pathogens, transmissible resistance genes are also found in the indigenous food microbiota such as lactobacilli or enterococci. Výrostková et al. [1] reported in their work that strains of *Lactobacillus johnsonii* from raw milk showed the highest resistance to erythromycin (34.8%), similar to *Lactobacillus zeae* (33.3%). Of the 41 isolates, the presence of an erythromycin-encoding transmissible gene was confirmed in five strains of *Lactobacillus johnsonii* and in two strains of *Lactobacillus zeae*, demonstrating the potential risk of spreading antimicrobial resistance through the food chain. Enterococci are often carriers of resistance genes that can also be transferred to other bacteria in food. A study by Lauková et al. [2] showed that enterococci in goat milk have moderate resistance to antibiotics but also low pathogenic potential, which could be used for the selection of potential probiotic strains. In addition, Hu et al. [3] stipulated that antimicrobial resistance of *Bacillus* spp. could be widespread in the food chain. It was reported that 57.9%, 26.3% and 21.5% of *Bacillus* strains (*B. cereus*, *B. licheniformis*, *B. pumilus* and *B. subtilis*) carried fosfomycin resistance gene *fosB*, tetracycline resistance gene *tet* and erythromycin resistance gene *erm*, respectively. The authors found a high rate of resistance of foodborne pathogen *B. cereus* from dairy products, including vancomycin-resistant strains carrying van genes detected by whole-genome sequencing.

Recently, great efforts have been made to study molds in food processing, food spoilage and food safety (mycotoxins). Molecular methods are being developed for their identification and better characterization in the food chain. Demjanová et al. [4] detected the mold species *Penicillium verrucosum*, *P. commune* and *P. crustosum* on the shell surfaces of table eggs using conventional polymerase chain reaction (PCR) and polymerase chain reaction-internal transcribed spacer restriction fragment length polymorphism method

(PCR-ITS-RFLP), confirming the presence of mycotoxin-producing strains and their importance for public health. Molecular identification of molds was performed in the study by Lešić et al. [5] focusing on the sensory properties of traditional fermented meat products. In the context of potential microbiological hazards, the authors reported that mycobiota were represented by a small proportion of mycotoxic mold species (12 and 14% in two types of dry-cured ham), identified as *Penicillium citrinum*, *Penicillium polonicum* and *Aspergillus niger*. In the work of Jevinová et al. [6], the effect of egg storage conditions on mold multiplication was studied. The authors reported that *Penicillium* and *Fusarium* species showed more intense growth with larger colony diameters on the eggshell surface at high relative humidity values, increasing the risk to consumers due to possible contamination of egg contents with mycotoxins. Interesting interactions among mold species were found in vitro, indicating the antifungal capacity of *Cladosporium cladoporioides* against *Penicillium chrysogenum*, *P. Crustosum* and *P. griseofulvum*.

The safety and quality characteristics of food can also be predicted by evaluating bacterial composition and growth during processing or storage. An example of this is the study by Kim et al. [7], in which metagenomic tools were used to correlate rancidity and microflora in dry-aged beef. Using analysis and quantification of microflora by qRT-PCR, the authors demonstrated that increases in the number of *Pantoea* spp. and decreases in the number of *Streptococcus* spp. could be used to determine rancidity of dry-aged beef and correlate with levels of reactive thiobarbituric acid (TBARS) and volatile basic nitrogen (VBN). In different cheese types, Zdolec et al. [8] demonstrated the effect of microbiota on biogenic amine content, focusing on applied bacterial or mold dairy cultures. The study showed that higher levels of biogenic amines, mainly tyramine, in cheeses were associated with the presence of *Enterococcus durans*, while negligible concentrations of amines were found in cheeses ripened with *Lacticaseibacillus rhamnosus*, *Lactococcus lactis* or *Lacticaseibacillus paracasei* cultures. The composition of the indigenous cheese microbiota was also investigated in the work of Lauková et al. [9] using next-generation sequencing. The results clearly confirmed the reliability of the method, revealing bacterial genera and their proportion in the population in a way that is not possible with traditional culturable methods.

The final review article in this Special Issue [10] presents a risk-based approach to ensuring meat safety from farm to slaughterhouse. It discusses the main biological hazards (bacteria, parasites) in the meat chain, focusing on under-controlled pathogens. On-farm food safety measures appear to be critical to reducing meatborne hazards and risk to consumers. Practical improvements in the control of biological hazards in the meat chain are still needed, and further developments can be expected in coming years.

As guest editor of the Special Issue "Study of Microbiological Safety in the Food Chain", I would like to thank all the authors, reviewers and supporting editors of the journal. I hope that this Special Issue will provide relevant new insights to scientists and professionals working in the field of food microbiology and public health.

Funding: This research received no external funding.

Acknowledgments: This work on the Special Issue was supported by the University of Zagreb, Faculty of Veterinary Medicine, and the projects "Potential of microencapsulation in cheese production" K.K.01.1.1.04.0058, funded by the EU Operational Programme Competitiveness and Cohesion 2014-2020 and "CEKOM 3LJ" K.K.01.2.2.03.0017 of the European Regional Development Fund.

Conflicts of Interest: The author declares no conflict of interest.

References

1. Výrostková, J.; Regecová, I.; Kováčová, M.; Marcinčák, S.; Dudriková, E.; Maľová, J. Antimicrobial Resistance of *Lactobacillus johnsonii* and *Lactobacillus zeae* in Raw Milk. *Processes* **2020**, *8*, 1627. [CrossRef]
2. Lauková, A.; Focková, V.; Pogány Simonová, M. Enterococcal Species Associated with Slovak Raw Goat Milk, Their Safety and Susceptibility to Lantibiotics and Durancin ED26E/7. *Processes* **2021**, *9*, 681. [CrossRef]

3. Hu, Q.; Fang, Y.; Zhu, J.; Xu, W.; Zhu, K. Characterization of *Bacillus* Species from Market Foods in Beijing, China. *Processes* **2021**, *9*, 866. [CrossRef]
4. Demjanová, S.; Jevinová, P.; Pipová, M.; Regecová, I. Identification of *Penicillium verrucosum*, *Penicillium commune*, and *Penicillium crustosum* Isolated from Chicken Eggs. *Processes* **2021**, *9*, 53. [CrossRef]
5. Lešić, T.; Vahčić, N.; Kos, I.; Zadravec, M.; Milićević, D.; Perković, I.; Listeš, E.; Pleadin, J. The Influence of Surface Mycobiota on Sensory Properties of "Istarski pršut" and "Dalmatinski pršut". *Processes* **2021**, *9*, 2287. [CrossRef]
6. Jevinová, P.; Pipová, M.; Regecová, I.; Demjanová, S.; Semjon, B.; Marcinčák, S.; Nagy, J.; Kožárová, I. Effect of *Cladosporium cladosporioides* on the Composition of Mycoflora and the Quality Parameters of Table Eggs during Storage. *Processes* **2021**, *9*, 613. [CrossRef]
7. Kim, S.; Kim, J.-C.; Park, S.; Kim, J.; Yoon, Y.; Lee, H. Identification of Microbial Flora in Dry Aged Beef to Evaluate the Rancidity during Dry Aging. *Processes* **2021**, *9*, 2049. [CrossRef]
8. Zdolec, N.; Bogdanović, T.; Severin, K.; Dobranić, V.; Kazazić, S.; Grbavac, J.; Pleadin, J.; Petričević, S.; Kiš, M. Biogenic Amine Content in Retailed Cheese Varieties Produced with Commercial Bacterial or Mold Cultures. *Processes* **2022**, *10*, 10. [CrossRef]
9. Lauková, A.; Micenková, L.; Pogány Simonová, M.; Focková, V.; Ščerbová, J.; Tomáška, M.; Dvorožňáková, E.; Košta, M. Microbiome Associated with Slovak Traditional Ewe's Milk Lump Cheese. *Processes* **2021**, *9*, 1603. [CrossRef]
10. Zdolec, N.; Kiš, M. Meat Safety from Farm to Slaughter—Risk-Based Control of *Yersinia enterocolitica* and *Toxoplasma gondii*. *Processes* **2021**, *9*, 815. [CrossRef]

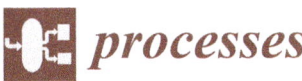

Review

Meat Safety from Farm to Slaughter—Risk-Based Control of *Yersinia enterocolitica* and *Toxoplasma gondii*

Nevijo Zdolec and Marta Kiš *

Department of Hygiene, Technology and Food Safety, Faculty of Veterinary Medicine, University of Zagreb, Heinzelova 55, 10000 Zagreb, Croatia; nzdolec@vef.hr
* Correspondence: mkis@vef.hr; Tel.: +38-51-239-0199

Abstract: The implementation of the traditional meat safety control system has significantly contributed to increasing food safety and public health protection. However, several biological hazards have emerged in meat production, requiring a comprehensive approach to their control, as traditional methods of meat inspection at the slaughterhouse are not able to detect them. While national control programs exist for the most important meat-related hazards, similar data are still lacking for certain neglected threats, such as *Yersinia enterocolitica* or *Toxoplasma gondii*. The obstacle in controlling these hazards in the meat chain is their presence in latently infected, asymptomatic animals. Their effective control can only be achieved through systematic preventive measures, surveillance or monitoring, and antimicrobial interventions on farms and in slaughterhouses. To establish such a system, it is important to collect all relevant data on hazard-related epidemiological indicators from the meat chain, which should provide relevant guidance for interventions at the harvest and post-harvest stage. The proposed approach is expected to improve the existing system and provide many opportunities to improve food safety and public health.

Keywords: meat safety; biological hazards; *Yersinia enterocolitica*; *Toxoplasma gondii*; food chain information

Citation: Zdolec, N.; Kiš, M. Meat Safety from Farm to Slaughter—Risk-Based Control of *Yersinia enterocolitica* and *Toxoplasma gondii*. *Processes* **2021**, *9*, 815. https://doi.org/10.3390/pr9050815

Academic Editor: José Manuel Moreno-Rojas

Received: 13 April 2021
Accepted: 5 May 2021
Published: 7 May 2021

Publisher's Note: MDPI stays neutral with regard to jurisdictional claims in published maps and institutional affiliations.

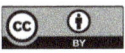

Copyright: © 2021 by the authors. Licensee MDPI, Basel, Switzerland. This article is an open access article distributed under the terms and conditions of the Creative Commons Attribution (CC BY) license (https://creativecommons.org/licenses/by/4.0/).

1. Introduction

Different husbandry systems of farm animals are burdened with specific biological and chemical hazards, which are transmitted throughout the meat production chain from the farm to the consumer [1]. In the past, appropriate preventive measures and control systems were developed on the basis of systematic hazard analyzes and designed according to epidemiological conditions at specific times. For example, at the beginning of veterinary controls on farm animal health and meat safety (19th century), controls were already risk-based and focused on zoonoses such as tuberculosis, cysticercosis, or trichinosis [2]. Nowadays, due to systematic controls and the implementation of veterinary and hygiene measures, these zoonoses occur less frequently and the risk is negligible [3]. However, this is not equally true for all parts of the world [4–7].

Recently, "new" biological hazards have emerged in livestock and meat production, requiring a comprehensive approach to their control and monitoring. These hazards existed before, but prevention and control measures did not comprehensively address them [8,9]. Specifically, the safety of meat is mainly threatened by the so-called invisible hazards, i.e., biological and chemical contaminants such as bacteria, viruses, parasites, toxins, residues of veterinary drugs, environmental contaminants, etc., which do not cause clinical symptoms or visible changes in the meat or animal organs [1]. Traditional methods of meat inspection in slaughterhouses are not able to detect these hazards, which requires a more risk-based approach to reduce the risk to public health [8,9]. Therefore, the main biological hazards in meat production, both at farm and slaughterhouse level, are *Salmonella* spp., *Campylobacter* spp., *Yersinia enterocolitica*, verotoxic *Escherichia coli*, bacteria with ESBL/AmpC gene, *Trichinella*, and *Toxoplasma gondii* [10]. The obstacle in controlling these hazards in the meat chain is their presence in latently infected, asymptomatic animals. As detection of these hazards on each individual carcass is impractical and unprofitable, their effective control is only possible through the application of a system of prevention and control measures on farms and in slaughterhouses [11,12].

In recent years, efforts have been made to establish a comprehensive integrated risk-based meat safety assurance system [9,13]. It is based on the identification of current public health risks and the implementation of control measures throughout the agri-food chain. In practice, this means that control and intervention measures are designed in slaughterhouses (harvest stage) according to previously identified hazards/risks on the farm (pre-harvest stage). The categorization of farms and slaughterhouses should help to better inform consumers about the level of safety on farms, which in turn may affect the practice of high-risk farms or slaughterhouses [9]. The categorization of farms and slaughter animals is based on food chain information (FCI) collected and recorded from the farm management system, surveillance, or monitoring programs and results of official controls [14,15]. These data guide the official veterinarian/risk manager in slaughterhouses when deciding on ante-mortem inspections, logistic slaughter, slaughter bans, visual or traditional meat inspection methods, decontamination procedures, and sampling for laboratory analysis. In the case of non-compliant data from the production chain on these hazards, risk reduction or elimination measures are chosen, such as decontamination of carcasses, freezing of meat, detailed post-mortem inspection, or additional laboratory testing [10,13]. Since the risk of bacterial pathogens in meat depends largely on the hygiene of the process between slaughterhouses [11], it is necessary to carry out risk categorization. In this way, improved meat safety is achieved in relation to the technology used in the slaughter process (Good Hygiene Practice, Good Manufacturing Practice) and, if necessary, the possibilities of decontamination technologies [11].

With regard to the listed priority biological hazards (pathogenic bacteria and parasites), the categorization of animals/farms should take into account the results of previous laboratory tests (if available) and adjust sampling and analysis plans according to trends [9,13]. Reliable data on certain prioritized threats, such as *Yersinia enterocolitica* or *Toxoplasma gondii* are still lacking at the farm/slaughterhouse level. The FCI needs to be complemented by Harmonized Epidemiological Indicators (HEIs), which provides the risk score of a specific part of the meat chain [14,15]. The purpose of this paper is to present the elements of a risk-based control system from farm to slaughterhouse, with a particular focus on *Y. enterocolitica* and *T. gondii* as examples of underestimated meat-borne hazards within the existing regulatory framework.

2. Biological Hazards in the Meat Chain

Bacterial intestinal pathogens have always been a challenge in meat hygiene, such as *Salmonella* spp., *Yersinia* spp., *Campylobacter* spp., *Listeria monocytogenes*, or *Escherichia coli* [1]. They are not physiologically present in the meat but get there during the slaughter processing of the animals, but also in the further course of handling and processing of meat by equipment, surfaces, and personnel [11,12]. Therefore, their finding on the meat (surface contamination) is due to their presence in slaughtered animals [1]. Recent systematic studies show that the prevalence of *Salmonella* and *Campylobacter* in broilers or pigs is over 20% and 50%, respectively, but it depends on the type of samples (from animals or the environment—the farm), the rearing method, and the area of observation (Table 1). The seroprevalence of *Y. enterocolitica* is highest in pigs and poses a greater meat safety challenge than *Salmonella* in some countries [15]. Shiga toxin-producing *E. coli* (STEC) has also shown an upward trend among foodborne zoonoses in recent years, but there are few data on its prevalence on farms. Regarding the results of national programs for the surveillance of specific pathogens of meat-borne diseases, such as in the EU, there are significantly lower prevalence compared to global/continental scientific studies (Table 2). The number of EU countries reporting the results of their on-farm bacterial surveillance programs is inconsistent and varies considerably across species. This is particularly true at the slaughter stage, where data are most complete only for *Salmonella* in pigs, and there are almost no data for the prevalence of *Yersinia* and STEC on carcasses of slaughtered animals (Table 3). Of the parasitic zoonoses, *Toxoplasma gondii* is considered a priority hazard in the meat production chain. This is supported by data on its high prevalence in pigs worldwide [16] and in ruminants and certain wildlife species [17]. National control programs exists for several prioritized meat-related hazards in many countries, but similar programs for *Y. enterocolitica* and *T. gondii* are missing [15].

Table 1. Recent studies on (sero)prevalence of main biological hazards in farm animals.

Animal Species	Biological Hazard	Sampling	Prevalence	Country, Reference
Broilers	*Salmonella* spp.	Environmental samples—boot sock, feces, litter, drag swab, feed, water, grass, soil, compost	22.9% (95% CI: 14.5–34.2%) and 19.9% (95% CI: 7.1–44.8%) for conventional and alternative samples, respectively	USA (systematic review), [18]
	Campylobacter spp.		15.8% (95% CI: 3–52%) and 52.8% (95% CI: 32.8–71.8%) for conventional and alternative samples, respectively	
Pigs, poultry, cattle, goat, sheep	*Salmonella* spp.	Gut samples	27.8% (95% CI 20.4–36.7); 40.2% (95% CI 32.7–48.2); 15.4% (95% CI 11.7–20.0); 16.8% (95% CI 11.4–24.6); 13.6% (95% CI 8.5–21.1)	Africa (systematic review), [19]
	Campylobacter spp.		15.4% (95% CI 8.4–26.6); 13.4% (95% CI 9.8–18.0); 4.5% (95% CI 2.9–6.9); 2.2% (95% CI 1.1–4.3); 4.5% (95% CI 2.8–7.2)	
Cattle	*Salmonella* spp.	Feces	9% (95% CI 7–11%)	Global (systematic review), [20]
Pigs	*Yersinia enterocolitica*	2353 meat juice samples, 259 farms	57% of pigs and 85% of farms	[15]
	Toxoplasma gondii		3% of pigs, 9% of farms	
Pigs	*Yersinia enterocolitica*	57 indoor fattening pig farms, serum	72.3%	[15]
	Toxoplasma gondii		<1%	
	Salmonella spp.		1.9–17.6%	
Pigs	*Toxoplasma gondii*	148,092 pigs from 47 countries	19% (95% CI: 17–22%)	Global (systematic review), [16]
Pigs, sheep, cattle, wild boars, moose	*Toxoplasma gondii*		6% in domestic pigs (CI 95%: 3–10%), 23% in sheep (CI 95%: 12–36%), 7% in cattle (CI 95%: 1–21%), 33% in wild boars (CI 95%: 26–41%), and 16% in moose (CI 95%: 10–23%)	Nordic-Baltic region in northern Europe (systematic review), [17]

Table 2. Official data on (sero)prevalence of main biological hazards in farm animal [21].

Biological Hazard	Animal Species	Sampling	Prevalence	Countries Reported the Data
Salmonella spp.	Broilers	National Control Programs, n = 361,974 flocks	3.48%, range by countries: 0–18.4%	29 EU countries
	Cattle	Feces, farm environmental samples; 25,687 cattle, 3962 herds	4.13% of animals and 0.88% of herds	13 EU countries
	Pigs	Caecum, feces, lymph nodes; 16,947 animals, 71,006 slaughter animal batch, 732 herds	0.97% in pigs, 53.2% in slaughter animal batch, 3.96% in herds	13 EU countries
Campylobacter spp.	Broilers	Caecum, n = 17,445 flocks/batch	22.18%	18 EU countries
	Turkey	Caecum, n = 1228	68.81%	5 EU countries
	Pigs	Feces, organs, n = 2504	2.12%	9 EU countries
	Cattle	Animal samples, n = 31,842	0.53%	12 EU countries
Yersinia enterocolitica	Pigs	Animal samples, n = 2354	0.43%	7 EU countries
	Domestic livestock other than pigs	Animal samples, n = 12,834	1.66%	6 EU countries
Toxoplasma gondii	Pigs	Blood, n = 263	22.05%	4 EU countries
	Sheep and goats	Blood, animal samples, n = 6818	5.47%	14 EU countries
	Cattle	Blood, animal samples, n = 159	27.7%	7 EU countries
STEC	Cattle	Feces, animal samples, n = 390	3.59%	2 EU countries
	Pigs	Feces, animal samples, n = 5	20%	2 EU countries
	Goats	Feces, animal samples, n = 5	40%	1 EU country

Table 3. Official data on prevalence of main biological hazards on carcasses at slaughter [21].

Biological Hazard	Animal Species	Sampling	Prevalence	Countries Reported the Data
Salmonella spp.	Broilers and turkey, chilled carcasses	Neck skin/carcass, n = 2381	15.08%	7 EU countries
	Cattle, sheep, goats and horses—carcasses before chilling	Carcass swabs 400 cm^2, n = 3848	0.55%	8 EU countries
	Pigs	Carcass swabs 100/400 cm^2, n = 149,962	1.62%	28 EU countries
Campylobacter spp.	Broilers, chilled carcasses	Neck skin/carcass, n = 3746 (PHC Reg. 2073)	35% (8.94% units with >1000 cfu)	10 EU countries
	Fresh broiler meat	1/10/25 g, n = 3621	27.9%	11 EU countries

Table 3. Cont.

Biological Hazard	Animal Species	Sampling	Prevalence	Countries Reported the Data
Yersinia enterocolitica	Pigs	Carcass swabs, n = 115	0.87%	1 EU country
STEC	Broilers	Carcass meat, 25 g, n = 31	22.58%	1 EU country
	Goats	Carcass swabs, 400 cm^2, n = 3	33.3%	1 EU country
	Horses, rabbits	Carcass swabs, 400 cm^2, n = 9	0.0%	1 EU country

3. Underestimated Biological Hazards in Meat Chain Control

3.1. Yersinia enterocolitica

Yersinia enterocolitica is an important and often neglected pathogenic microorganism in veterinary public health and meat hygiene [12]. Human yersiniosis is one of the leading foodborne zoonoses and has been declared as the fourth zoonosis after campylobacteriosis, salmonellosis, and Shiga toxin-producing *E. coli* infection, according to EU data [21]. Although bacterial transmission to humans usually occurs through raw or undercooked food or water, some infections have been reported under the low level of personal hygiene [12,15]. Infection with pathogenic *Y. enterocolitica* is usually manifested by milder gastrointestinal symptoms that usually do not require treatment. Therefore, the actual number of infected individuals is believed to be much higher than the number of reported cases, so that the public health importance of this bacterium has been underestimated over time [12].

3.1.1. Farm Risk Factors and Serological Testing

Domestic pigs are the most important carriers of pathogenic *Y. enterocolitica* strains as well as a source of contamination of meat intended for human consumption [12]. At the farm level, it is estimated that pathogen prevalence is higher in conventional intensive farming systems than in organic extensive farming systems [22] and may be seasonal [23]. Regarding the colonization and occurrence of *Y. enterocolitica* in different categories of pigs, most studies indicate persistence of the risk in fattening pigs. Fecal shedding of pathogens begins at one to three months of age and peaks at two to five months of age. After this age, fecal incidence decreases, but pigs remain seropositive for a longer period of time [24]. It is estimated that 35–70% of swine herds and 45–100% of individual finishing pigs are carriers of *Y. enterocolitica* [25]. Our recent study (unpublished) showed that despite the same (highest) biosecurity levels in integrated pig farms, the prevalence of pathogenic *Y. enterocolitica* was significantly different between farms, suggesting that risk factors for the occurrence of the pathogen in tonsils may be related to harvest level [26]. In contrast to integrated farming systems, a significant influence of biosecurity level on pathogen prevalence was found in small family farms, i.e., the lower the biosecurity level of the farm, the higher the pathogen prevalence [26].

In terms of risk factors, Virtanen et al. [27] found that infection (carrier status) and excretion of *Y. enterocolitica* in feces was prevented by the use of municipal water, purchase of pig feed from a single trusted supplier and organic production (i.e., protective factor). The risk factors for the excretion of *Y. enterocolitica* in feces are carrier status of the pathogen on tonsils, purchase of pig feed from multiple suppliers, feeding pigs before transport to slaughterhouse, and snout contact. Vilar et al. [28] also claim that the prevalence of *Y. enterocolitica* in pigs can be reduced by using only municipal water and an all-in/all-out system, while a lack of bedding and the purchase of piglets from multiple farms are risk factors.

To categorize farms in terms of *Yersinia* risk, the use of serological monitoring prior to slaughter has been strongly recommended in recent years [29]. Felin et al. [30] reported strong correlation between seropositivity to *Salmonella* and *Yersinia* in fattening pigs. Moreover, the housing system was also important factor for *Yersinia* seroprevalence [30]. Serological results in FCI give the possibility for the slaughterhouse to risk-rank farms according to the risk of shedding *Yersinia*, and slaughter the pigs from high-risk farms at the end of the day and use hot water decontamination for these carcasses [15].

3.1.2. Prevalence of Pathogen in Pigs

Pigs are asymptomatic carriers of strains pathogenic to humans, mainly biotype 4 (serotype O:3) and less frequently biotype 2 (serotype O:9 and O:5.27). They are found in the oral cavity, particularly in the tonsils, submandibular lymph nodes, tongue, and intestines and feces [31]. It is common to find strains of bioserotype 4/O:3 on the surface of slaughtered carcasses due to fecal contamination, intestinal, and tonsil contents during slaughter processing [32]. The detection of *Y. enterocolitica* in the tonsils depends on numerous factors, such as the time of infection (on-farm, during transport, in the slaughterhouse barn) or slaughterhouse practices (cross-contamination). For example, the procedures during housing before slaughter are very important for the spread of pathogens between groups of pigs in lairage [29]. Nowak et al. [33] recorded a higher prevalence of *Y. enterocolitica*, particularly in the tonsils, in pigs slaughtered at the end of the day than in pigs slaughtered at the beginning. This suggests the contamination of pigs brought to slaughter from different sources, and contamination occurred via feces from previously dormant pigs in the herd. Indeed, after oral infection, the bacteria can be detected in the appendix and lymph nodes within only three hours [29,33].

The prevalence of *Y. enterocolitica* in the tonsils of slaughtered pigs varies widely in Europe, ranging from 1.8 to 93% [34,35]. The highest recovery rate of the pathogen is found in tonsils, and it is lower in intestines or on pig carcasses. In the UK, the prevalence of *Y. enterocolitica* in tonsils was 28.7%, while in carcasses, it was only 1.8% [36]. In Belgian slaughterhouses, 55.1% of tonsil samples, 25.1% of fecal samples, and 39.1% of carcasses were positive. The incidence of the pathogens was highest in the tonsil region (29%) and much lower in the pelvic and sternum regions (7–16%) [37]. Centorame et al. [38] reported a relatively low prevalence of 9.31% in the tonsils, but the dominance of bioserotype 4/O:3 (95.74%) indicates the importance of pigs as natural reservoirs for human yersiniosis. In Brazil, a prevalence of 25.2% was reported from pig tonsils with only two pathogenic strains, confirming high variability in pathogen persistence between countries [39]. In a Croatian study [32], *Y. enterocolitica* bioserotype 4/O:3 strains were recovered from 33.3% of tonsils and 10.25% of mandibular lymph nodes. A recent study from the same pig farming system and slaughterhouses in Croatia revealed a prevalence of 43% of pathogenic *Y. enterocolitica* 4/O:3 in pig tonsils [26]. The above survey reports indicate high variability in prevalence between studies, which is possibly due to differences in farm management, sampling methods, hygienic practices at slaughter, and, in particular, methods of pathogen isolation and detection.

3.1.3. Meat Contamination at Slaughter and Meat Processing

Regarding the risk of meat contamination during slaughter, Vilar et al. [28] claim that the presence of *Y. enterocolitica* in the intestines, tonsils, and offal are the main risk factors, which also leads to a higher probability of cross-contamination. The prevention of meat contamination during slaughter should be based on standard operative procedures such as bunging/rectum tying and removal of the head together with the tonsils [40]. Removal of the tonsils is a critical step as, for example, the parts of the tonsils remaining in the throat after evisceration can be a major cause of the spread of pathogens from lymphatic to muscle tissue [32,41,42]. It is also suggested to partially remove the viscera by leaving the tongue and tonsils on the halves and omitting the incision of the mandibular lymph nodes. In countries such as Denmark and Canada, carcass halves are decontaminated with hot water or steam to reduce the incidence of *Y. enterocolitica* [43].

With regard to slaughter techniques and possible failures in processing hygiene, contamination with pathogens is expected to occur mainly in the meat of the neck, head, tongue and throat region, less so in the carcass [44,45]. Martins et al. [46] isolated *Y. enterocolitica* from the tonsils and lymph nodes of pigs but not from the environmental samples or from the meat after carcass splitting. However, the presence of pathogenic *Y. enterocolitica*, even in low numbers, is a risk factor for consumers because of its ability to grow at lower temperatures, as well as temperature abuse during chilling [47,48]. In this regard, minced meat, characterized by high microbiological risk, is a possible source of *Y. enterocolitica* [49]. Visnubhatla et al. [50] recorded a high level of contamination of minced beef and pork with the pathogen *Y. enterocolitica* up to 6 log CFU/g, which poses a risk to the consumer. Recently, Ferl et al. [51] reported *Y. enterocolitica* contamination in minced pork (22.6%, N = 62) and seasoned minced meat (11.5%). Similarly, studies from Argentina, India, or Malesia indicate a higher prevalence of pathogenic *Y. enterocolitica* in fresh pork products on the market, but these results are highly variable and depend on risk factors such as the hygiene level of slaughter or farming practices [52–54].

3.2. Toxoplasma gondii

Toxoplasmosis is a worldwide zoonosis and one of the most common meat-borne parasitic diseases [12,16]. Recently, Aguirre et al. [55] presented the One Health approach to toxoplasmosis, which is one of the leading causes of death in the USA and has a high seroprevalence in humans (up to 90% in countries with low sanitary measures) [55]. Humans can become infected with the parasite via ingestion of oocysts directly from soil or in contaminated food or water; via ingestion of tissue cysts in uncooked/raw infected meat; or vertically from mother to child during primary infection in pregnancy [56]. However, it is known that consumption of undercooked meat is the most important factor [57]. In Europe, pork is generally considered the main source of invasions, while studies in Norway and France have shown that lamb is a more significant risk factor [58]. However, there is no official requirement for surveillance or control of *T. gondii* in meat-producing animals. Given the high prevalence and public health importance of *T. gondii*, it is necessary to establish an effective system to control this zoonosis in the meat production chain [12,16]. In the first place, the prevention of toxoplasmosis should be based on comprehensive control at the level of primary production (farm) and at the slaughterhouse, together with deactivation processes in meat processing [13]. To improve food safety, the European Food Safety Authority (EFSA) recommends the review of biosecurity measures in conventional finishing farms and serology in different types of herds to identify high-risk farms and use them within food chain information system [10,58].

3.2.1. Serological Testing—Pre-Harvest Control

The global seroprevalence of toxoplasmosis in pigs is estimated to 19%, and it is higher in free ranged systems [16]. Contrary, seroprevalence is lowest in intensive pig farming [59]. Serological methods are considered the primary method for diagnosing toxoplasmosis because it is asymptomatic in pigs and the cysts are too small to be detected during meat inspection at the slaughterhouse. To date, serological tests are regularly used to detect exposure in pigs and seroprevalence in general, both in pigs and other animals and in humans [12]. Serological testing for porcine toxoplasmosis in a slaughterhouse has proven to be the most practical method to obtain risk data from the farm and to take further control measures accordingly [15]. In particular, EFSA recommends serological testing of fattening pigs kept in uncontrolled housing systems [43].

Serology can only be used to assess the risk of infection to humans if there is a correlation between seroprevalence and the presence of cysts in meat. Opsteegh et al. [60] investigated this correlation for major domestic animal species and estimated that the probability of detection of parasites in seropositive animals was highest in pigs (58.8%), followed by chickens (53.4%), sheep, and goats (39.4% and 35.0%), and it was the lowest in horses and cattle. These data suggest that the correlation between antibody detection against *T. gondii* and direct parasite detection is high in pigs, small ruminants, and chickens. In these species, the use of serology can help determine the risk to the consumer, but it may not be as useful in other species, such as horses and cattle. In addition, a seronegative result does not necessarily mean that the meat is free of *T. gondii*. Therefore, an integrated approach combining serology with molecular techniques would provide a multilevel understanding of the epidemiology of the parasite, as molecular detection provides additional information on the risk of meat consumption [61]. In studies by Jurankova et al. [62], the brain, heart, and lungs were the preferred sites for *T. gondii* cysts in experimentally infected pigs.

Different serological methods were used to detect IgG antibodies in pig serum and meat juice. Meat juice is commonly used because it is readily available at slaughter and can also be used to detect other zoonotic diseases such as salmonellosis, yersiniosis, and trichinosis [43]. It should be noted that IgG antibody levels are lower in meat juice compared to serum, so it is necessary to use a lower dilution factor for meat juice samples. Antibodies usually persist until the time of slaughter [63], but the immune response cannot be measured immediately after infection. Sometimes, an animal's immune system is unable to produce a measurable immune response despite carrying a pathogen. Therefore, serological methods are not always suitable for testing individual carcasses as part of a food safety assessment [16,29,30]. However, Felin et al. [15] investigated the seroprevalence of fattening pigs for *T. gondii* to assess the feasibility of serological surveillance in the slaughterhouse and the usability of the results as part of the FCI. Although the seroprevalence of *T. gondii* was generally low, some farms were found with 100% seroprevalence. Serological surveillance in this case would allow the identification of farms where existing biosecurity measures should be introduced and improved. These farms should be visited and advised by veterinarians to improve biosecurity measures, reduce risk, and increase the safety of meat for consumers. Carcasses of pigs from such high-risk holdings should be frozen or subjected to heat treatment [12].

3.2.2. Controls at the Slaughterhouse and during Meat Processing

Toxoplasma gondii is considered a priority risk in meat inspection of pigs, farmed game (wild boar, deer), sheep, and goats [12]. It is impossible to detect the risk of *T. gondii* through the traditional way of inspection in slaughterhouses [10]; therefore, additional (pre-)testing in the meat chain is needed. Based on the collected data on the hazards in the production chain (e.g., serological testing of animals), the necessary measures are selected to reduce or eliminate the risks in the meat production chain, such as heat treatment and freezing of meat [64].

Several processing methods can be used to decontaminate meat containing bradyzoites of *T. gondii* [65]. Heat treatment is the safest method to inactivate the parasite [66]. It is recommended to cook pork at a temperature of 70 °C, and the meat should be cooked thoroughly until the internal temperature reaches 66 °C. Cooking temperature and avoidance of cross-contamination are considered the most important factors in preventing *T. gondii* infection from meat consumption [63]. Both cooking temperature and bradysoite concentration of *T. gondii* in muscle are the highest risk factors for transmission to humans [67]. Most cysts are inactivated by temperatures below -12 °C/2 days [13]. Gamma radiation has the same effect as high pressure treatment at 300 MPa or more [68]. The problem may be the effect of these methods on the color, texture, and flavor of the meat and therefore may be unattractive to the consumer. In addition, the use of gamma radiation and high-pressure processing may be restricted by legislation and may incur high costs [69]. As for cured meat products, most studies suggest that cysts of *T. gondii* are destroyed during salt curing, but the inactivation of these cysts depends on the maturation time, temperature of storage, and salt concentration in the curing process [70–73].

4. Food Chain Information and Epidemiological Indicators

A central role in the meat safety system is played by food chain information, which should provide relevant guidance for the management of a group of animals or a herd in relation to the prioritized biological hazards [12]. The usual information on health, drug treatment, nutrition, operational measures, etc. in the above context of the meat inspection system is not sufficient as it does not cover all the hazards and control measures discussed before, e.g., for *T. gondii* or *Y. enterocolitica* [15]. When carrying out inspection procedures, the official veterinarian shall take into account the certificates and attestations accompanying the animals and any declarations made by the veterinarian, including official and authorized veterinarians who have carried out controls at the level of primary production [2,3,15]. This information should help to increase food safety for consumers, as it would act as a link between the farm and the slaughterhouse [10].

However, in most European countries, there are currently no regular monitoring programs for the main meat-borne zoonoses on farms, except for salmonellosis in chicken broilers, turkey broilers, commercial chicken flocks, turkey and chicken breeding flocks and strains of *S.* Enteritidis, *S.* Typhimurium, *S.* Hadar, *S.* Infantis, and *S.* Virchow, in breeding flocks of chickens [21]. If these data from primary production are credible, complete, and applicable, they can greatly reduce the risk and hazards, i.e., increase the level of food safety [15]. Therefore, the categorization of risks in certain stages of production from farm to slaughterhouse should be enabled by Harmonized Epidemiological Indicators (HEIs) [12–14]. Thus, the risk of herds/flocks on the farm in terms of microbiological hazards can be assessed by monitoring the audit of the animal procurement system, monitoring husbandry practices and the presence/absence of target bacteria in the feces of the animals [12].

Monitoring of transport of slaughter animals and housing conditions at the slaughterhouse prior to slaughter provides information on the risk of a particular group of animals (batch). During slaughter processing, the risk is assessed by the bacteriological status of the carcass before and after skinning and before chilling. By microbiological testing after carcass chilling, we obtain data on the performance of the system in relation to the set targets (microbiological criteria for specific bacteria) on the carcass [9–13]. Accordingly, low-risk animals in relation to e.g., *Yersinia* are handled on a standard slaughter line that has a proven ability to ensure the achievement of carcass targets (e.g., absence of *Yersinia*) through good hygiene and production practices and the HACCP system. On the other hand, carcasses of animals from high-risk farms (e.g., seropositive to *Yersinia*) should be subjected to a decontamination process (steam, hot water) at the end of the slaughter line to reduce the potential risk. Where the risk of *Toxoplasma* is high, measures should include thermal treatment of the meat [9–13].

5. Conclusions

Nowadays, meat hygiene is confronted with new threats, making the veterinary profession even more important in the context of an integrated system for ensuring meat safety and a risk-based approach to official controls. In order to identify health risks, a comprehensive approach to meat production and inspection must incorporate knowledge of primary meat production and hygiene and all available information from the entire production system. In a safety assessment of meat, it is important to analyze data on the food chain (FCI), epidemiological indicators, herd health, animal welfare, and hygiene practices in slaughterhouses/farms. In this context, the importance of veterinarians at farm level is obvious, as is the flow of food chain information from farm to slaughterhouse and vice versa. Meat inspection is a logical extension with preventive measures and controls in primary production. However, even perfect management and prevention in primary production cannot guarantee reduced risk if hygiene and processing practices in slaughterhouses are poor. For both *Y. enterocolitica* and *T. gondii*, the control strategy should be based on epidemiological indicators and consequent intervention protocols to ensure safe meat for human consumption.

Author Contributions: Conceptualization, N.Z.; writing—original draft preparation, M.K.; writing—review and editing, N.Z. All authors have read and agreed to the published version of the manuscript.

Funding: This research received no external funding.

Institutional Review Board Statement: Not applicable.

Informed Consent Statement: Not applicable.

Data Availability Statement: Data is contained within the article.

Conflicts of Interest: The authors declare no conflict of interest.

References

1. Sofos, J.N. Challenges to meat safety in the 21st century. *Meat. Sci.* **2008**, *78*, 3–13. [CrossRef] [PubMed]
2. Edwards, D.S.; Johnston, M.; Mead, G.C. Meat Inspection: An Overview of Present Practices and Future Trends. *Vet. J.* **1997**, *154*, 135–147. [CrossRef]
3. Ries, L.E.; Hoelzer, K. Implementation of Visual-Only Swine Inspection in the European Union: Challenges, Opportunities, and Lessons Learned. *J. Food Protect.* **2020**, *83*, 1918–1928. [CrossRef]
4. Zdolec, N.; Vujević, I.; Dobranić, V.; Juras, M.; Grgurević, N.; Ardalić, D.; Njari, B. Prevalence of Cysticercus bovis in slaughtered cattle determined by traditional meat inspection in Croatian abattoir from 2005 to 2010. *Helminthologia* **2012**, *49*, 229–232. [CrossRef]
5. Ng-Nguyen, D.; Stevenson, M.A.; Traub, R.J. A systematic review of taeniasis, cysticercosis and trichinellosis in Vietnam. *Parasit. Vectors* **2017**, *10*, 1–15. [CrossRef] [PubMed]
6. Trevisan, C.; Sotiraki, S.; Laranjo-Gonzáles, M.; Dermauw, V.; Wang, Z.; Kärssin, A.; Cvetkovikj, A.; Winkler, A.S.; Abraham, A.; Bobić, B.; et al. Epidemiology of taeniosis/cysticercosis in Europe, a systematic review: Eastern Europe. *Parasit. Vectors* **2018**, *11*, 1–11, . [CrossRef]
7. Eichenberger, R.M.; Thomas, L.F.; Gabriël, S.; Bobić, B.; Devleesschauwer, B.; Robertson, L.J.; Saratsis, A.; Torgerson, P.R.; Braae, U.C.; Dermauw, V.; et al. Epidemiology of Taenia saginata taeniosis/cysticercosis: A systematic review of the distribution in East, Southeast and South Asia. *Parasit. Vectors* **2020**, *13*, 1–11. [CrossRef]
8. Alban, L.; Petersen, J.V.; Bækbo, A.K.; Østergaard Pedersen, T.; Kruse, A.B.; Pacheco, G.; Halberg Larsen, M. Modernising meat inspection of pigs—A review of the Danish process from 2006-2020. *Food Control* **2021**, *119*, 1–11. [CrossRef]
9. Blagojević, B.; Nesbakken, T.; Alvseike, O.; Vågsholm, I.; Antic, D.; Johlerf, S.; Houf, K.; Meemken, D.; Nastasijevic, I.; Vieira Pinto, M.; et al. Drivers, opportunities, and challenges of the European risk-based meat safety assurance system. *Food Control* **2021**, *124*, 1–12. [CrossRef]
10. Nastasijević, I.; Vesković, S.; Milijašević, M. Meat safety: Risk based assurance systems and novel technologies. *Meat Technol.* **2020**, *61*, 97. [CrossRef]
11. Blagojević, B.; Antić, D. Assessment of potential contribution of official meat inspection and abattoir process hygiene to biological safety assurance of final beef and pork carcasses. *Food Control* **2014**, *36*, 174–182. [CrossRef]
12. Ninios, T.; Lundén, J.; Korkeala, H.; Fredriksson-Ahomaa, M. *Meat Inspection and Control in the Slaughterhouse*; John Wiley & Sons: Oxford, UK, 2014.
13. Bunčić, S.; Alban, L.; Blagojević, B. From traditional meat inspection to development of meat safety assurance programs in pig abattoirs—The European situation. *Food Control* **2019**, *106*, 1–12. [CrossRef]
14. Gomes-Neves, E.; Muller, A.; Correia, A.; Capas-Peneda, S.; Carvalho, M.; Vieira, S.; Fonseca Cardoso, M. Food Chain Information: Data Quality and Usefulness in Meat Inspection in Portugal. *J. Food Protect.* **2018**, *81*, 1890–1896, . [CrossRef] [PubMed]
15. Felin, E. Towards Risk-Based Meat Inspection: Prerequisites of Risk-Based Meat Inspection of Pigs in Finland. Ph.D. Thesis, University of Helsinki, Helsinki, Finland, June 2019.
16. Foroutan, M.; Fakhric, Y.; Riahid, S.M.; Ebrahimpoure, S.; Namroodif, S.; Taghipourb, A.; Spoting, A.; Gamblei, H.R.; Rostami, A. The global seroprevalence of *Toxoplasma gondii* in pigs: A systematic review and meta-analysis. *Vet. Parasitol.* **2019**, *269*, 42–52. [CrossRef] [PubMed]
17. Olsen, A.; Berg, R.; Tagel, M.; Must, K.; Deksne, G.; Larsen Enemark, H.; Alban, L.; Vang Johansen, M.; Vedel Nielsen, H.; Sandberg, M.; et al. Seroprevalence of *Toxoplasma gondii* in domestic pigs, sheep, cattle, wild boars, and moose in the Nordic-Baltic region: A systematic review and meta-analysis. *Parasite Epidemiol. Control* **2019**, *3*, 1–13, . [CrossRef]
18. Golden, C.E.; Mishra, A. Prevalence of *Salmonella* and *Campylobacter* spp. in Alternative and Conventionally Produced Chicken in the United States: A Systematic Review and Meta-Analysis. *J. Food Protect.* **2020**, *83*, 1181–1197, . [CrossRef]
19. Thomas, K.M.; de Glanville, W.A.; Barker, G.C.; Benschop, J.; Buza, J.J.; Cleaveland, S.; Davis, M.A.; French, N.P.; Mmbaga, B.T.; Prinsen, G.; et al. Prevalence of *Campylobacter* and *Salmonella* in African food animals and meat: A systematic review and meta-analysis. *Int. J. Food Microbiol.* **2020**, *315*, 1–22, . [CrossRef]
20. Gutema, F.D.; Agga, G.E.; Abdi, R.D.; De Zutter, L.; Duchateau, L.; Gabriël, S. Prevalence and Serotype Diversity of *Salmonella* in Apparently Healthy Cattle: Systematic Review and Meta-Analysis of Published Studies, 2000-2017. *Front. Vet. Sci.* **2019**, *6*, 1–11. [CrossRef]

21. EFSA. The European union one health 2018 zoonoses report. *EFSA J.* **2019**, *17*, 1–275, . [CrossRef]
22. Laukkanen, R.; Martínez, P.O.; Siekkinen, K.M.; Ranta, J.; Maijala, R.; Korkeala, H. Contamination of Carcasses with Human Pathogenic *Yersinia enterocolitica* 4/O:3 Originates from Pigs Infected on Farms. *Foodborne Pathog. Dis.* **2009**, *6*, 681–688, . [CrossRef]
23. Fondrevez, M.; Minvielle, B.; Labbé, A.; Houdayer, C.; Rose, N.; Esnault, E.; Denis, M. Prevalence of pathogenic *Yersinia enterocolitica* in slaughter-aged pigs during a one-year survey, 2010-2011, France. *Int. J. Food Microbiol.* **2014**, *174*, 56–62, . [CrossRef] [PubMed]
24. Koskinen, J.; Keto-Timonen, R.; Virtanen, S.; Vilar, M.J.; Korkeala, H. Prevalence and Dynamics of Pathogenic *Yersinia enterocolitica* 4/O:3 Among Finnish Piglets, Fattening Pigs and Sows. *Foodborne Pathog. Dis.* **2019**, *16*, 831–839, . [CrossRef]
25. Shoaib, M.; Shehzad, A.; Raza, H.; Niazi, S.; Khan, I.M.; Akhtar, W.; Safdar, W.; Wang, Z. A comprehensive review on the prevalence, pathogenesis and detection of *Yersinia enterocolitica*. *RSC Adv.* **2019**, *9*, 41010–41021. [CrossRef]
26. Pažin, V. Phenotypic and genetic characteristics of Yersinia enterocolitica isolated from pork production chain. Unpublished.
27. Virtanen, S.E.; Salonen, L.K.; Laukkanen, R.; Hakkinen, M.; Korkeala, H. Factors related to the prevalence of pathogenic *Yersinia enterocolitica* on pig farms. *Epidemiol. Infect.* **2011**, *139*, 1919–1927, . [CrossRef]
28. Vilar, M.J.; Virtanen, S.; Laukkanen-Ninios, R.; Korkeala, H. Bayesian modelling to identify the risk factors for *Yersinia enterocolitica* contamination of pork carcasses and pluck sets in slaughterhouses. *Int. J. Food Microbiol.* **2015**, *197*, 53–57, . [CrossRef] [PubMed]
29. Bonardi, S.; Bruini, I.; D'incau, M.; Van Damme, I.; Carniel, E.; Brémont, S.; Cavallini, P.; Tagliabue, S.; Brindani, F. Detection, seroprevalence and antimicrobial resistance of *Yersinia enterocolitica* and *Yersinia pseudotuberculosis* in pig tonsils in Northern Italy. *Int. J. Food Microbiol.* **2016**, *235*, 125–132, . [CrossRef]
30. Felin, E.; Jukola, E.; Raulo, S.; Fredriksson-Ahomaa, M. Meat Juice Serology and Improved Food Chain Information as Control Tools for Pork-Related Public Health Hazards. *Zoonoses Public Health* **2014**, *62*, 456–464. [CrossRef] [PubMed]
31. Moreira, L.M.; Milan, C.; Gonçalves, T.G.; Nunes Ebersol, C.; Gonzales de Lima, H.; Timm, C.D. Contamination of pigs by *Yersinia enterocolitica* in the abattoir flowchart and its relation to the farm. *Ciênc. Rural* **2019**, *49*, 1–7. [CrossRef]
32. Zdolec, N.; Dobranić, V.; Filipović, I. Prevalence of *Salmonella* spp. and *Yersinia enterocolitica* in/on tonsils and mandibular lymph nodes of slaughtered pigs. *Folia Microbiol.* **2015**, *60*, 131–135. [CrossRef] [PubMed]
33. Nowak, B.; Mueffling, T.V.; Caspari, K.; Hartung, J. Validation of a method for the detection of virulent *Yersinia enterocolitica* and their distribution in slaughter pigs from conventional and alternative housing systems. *Vet. Microbiol.* **2006**, *117*, 219–228, . [CrossRef] [PubMed]
34. O'Sullivan, T.; Friendship, R.; Blackwell, T.; Pearl, D.; McEwen, B.; Carman, S.; Slavić, Đ.; Dewey, C. Microbiological identification and analysis of swine tonsils collected from carcasses at slaughter. *Can. J. Vet. Res.* **2011**, *75*, 106–111.
35. Martínez, P.O.; Fredriksson-Ahomaa, M.; Pallotti, A.; Rosmini, R.; Houf, K.; Korkeala, H. Variation in the Prevalence of Enteropathogenic *Yersinia* in Slaughter Pigs from Belgium, Italy, and Spain. *Foodborne Pathog. Dis.* **2011**, *8*, 445–450. [CrossRef]
36. Powell, L.F.; Cheney, T.E.A.; Williamson, S.; Guy, E.; Smith, R.P.; Davies, R.H. A prevalence study of *Salmonella* spp., *Yersinia* spp., *Toxoplasma gondii* and porcine reproductive and respiratory syndrome virus in UK pigs at slaughter. *Epidemiol. Infect.* **2015**, *144*, 1538–1549. [CrossRef]
37. Van Damme, I.; Berkvens, D.; Vanantwerpen, G.; Baré, J.; Houf, K.; Wauters, G.; De Zutter, L. Contamination of freshly slaughtered pig carcasses with enteropathogenic *Yersinia* spp.: Distribution, quantification and identification of risk factors. *Int. J. Food Microbiol.* **2015**, *204*, 33–40. [CrossRef] [PubMed]
38. Centorame, P.; Sulli, N.; De Fanis, C.; Colangelo, O.V.; De Massis, F.; Conte, A.; Persiani, T.; Marfoglia, C.; Scattolini, S.; Pomilio, F.; et al. Identification and characterization of *Yersinia enterocolitica* strains isolated from pig tonsils at slaughterhouse in Central Italy. *Vet. Ital.* **2017**, *53*, 331–344. [CrossRef] [PubMed]
39. Wildemann, P.; Gava, D.; Pilegi Sfaciotte, R.A.; Melo, F.D.; Ferraz, S.M.; da Costa, U.M.; Vaz, E.K. Low occurrence of pathogenic *Yersinia enterocolitica* in pig tonsils at slaughter in Southern Brazil. *Trop. Anim. Health Prod.* **2017**, *50*, 671–675. [CrossRef] [PubMed]
40. Laukkanen, R.; Ranta, J.; Dong, X.; Hakkinen, M.; Martínez, P.O.; Lundén, J.; Johansson, T.; Korkeala, H. Reduction of Enteropathogenic *Yersinia* in the Pig Slaughterhouse by Using Bagging of the Rectum. *J. Food Protect.* **2010**, *73*, 2161–2168. [CrossRef]
41. Nesbakken, T.; Eckner, K.; Høidal, H.K.; Røtterud, O.J. Occurrence of *Yersinia enterocolitica* and *Campylobacter* spp. in slaughter pigs and consequences for meat inspection, slaughtering and dressing procedures. *Int. J. Food Microbiol.* **2003**, *80*, 231–240. [CrossRef]
42. Bonardi, S.; Alpigiani, I.; Pongolini, S.; Morganti, M.; Tagliabue, S.; Bacci, C.; Briandini, F. Detection, enumeration and characterization of *Yersinia enterocolitica* 4/O:3 in pig tonsils at slaughter in Northern Italy. *Int. J. Food Microbiol.* **2014**, *177*, 9–15. [CrossRef]
43. Fredriksson-Ahomaa. Yersinia enterocolitica. In *Foodborne Diseases*, 3rd ed.; Dodd, C.E.R., Aldsworth, T., Stein, R.A., Cliver, D.O., Riemann, H.P., Eds.; Academic Press: London, UK, 2017; pp. 223–232.
44. Messelhäusser, U.; Kämpf, P.; Colditz, J.; Bauer, H.; Schreiner, H.; Höller, C.; Busch, U. Qualitative and Quantitative Detection of Human Pathogenic *Yersinia enterocolitica* in Different Food Matrices at Retail Level in Bavaria. *Foodborne Pathog. Dis.* **2011**, *8*, 39–44. [CrossRef]

45. Laukkanen-Ninios, R.; Fredriksson-Ahomaa, M.; Maijala, R.; Korkeala, H. High prevalence of pathogenic *Yersinia enterocolitica* in pig cheeks. *Food Microbiol.* **2014**, *43*, 50–52. [CrossRef]
46. Martins, B.T.F.; Botelho, C.V.; Lopes Silva, D.A.; Lanna, F.G.P.A.; Libero Grossi, J.; Campos-Galvão, M.E.M.; Seiti Yamatogi, R.; Pfrimer Falcão, J.; dos Santos Bersot, L.; Nero, L.A. *Yersinia enterocolitica* in a Brazilian pork production chain: Tracking of contamination routes, virulence and antimicrobial resistance. *Int. J. Food Microbiol.* **2018**, *276*, 5–9. [CrossRef]
47. Bijelić, T.; Dobranić, V.; Kazazić, S.; Filipović, I.; Dumbović, Z.; Zdolec, N. Growth of *Yersinia enterocolitica* O:3 in minced pork meat. *Vet. Stn.* **2017**, *48*, 25–29.
48. Vujić, K.; Kiš, M.; Zdolec, N. Microbial contamination of food refrigerators in households. *Veterinar* **2020**, *58*, 23–27.
49. Fredriksson-Ahomaa, M.; Korkeala, H. Molecular epidemiology of *Yersinia enterocolitica* 4/O:3. In *The Genus Yersinia*; Skurnik, M., Bengoechea, J.A., Granfors, K., Eds.; Springer: New York, NY, USA, 2003; pp. 295–302.
50. Vishnubhatla, A.; Oberst, R.D.; Fung, D.Y.C.; Wonglumsom, W.; Hays, M.P.; Nagaraja, T.G. Evaluation of a 5′-nuclease (TaqMan) Assay for the Detection of Virulent Strains of *Yersinia enterocolitica* in Raw Meat and Tofu Samples. *J. Food Protect.* **2001**, *64*, 355–360, . [CrossRef]
51. Ferl, M.; Mäde, D.; Braun, P.G. Combined molecular biological and microbiological detection of pathogenic *Yersinia enterocolitica* in spiced ground pork, meat for production of ground pork and raw sausages. *JVL* **2020**, *15*, 27–35. [CrossRef]
52. Lucero-Estrada, C.S.M.; Soria, J.M.; Favier, G.I.; Escudero, M.E. Evaluation of the pathogenic potential, antimicrobial susceptibility and genomic relations of *Yersinia enterocolitica* strains from food and human origin. *Can. J. Microbiol.* **2015**, *61*, 851–860, . [CrossRef]
53. Latha, C.; Anu, C.J.; Ajaykumar, V.J.; Sunil, B. Prevalence of *Listeria monocytogenes, Yersinia enterocolitica, Staphylococcus aureus,* and *Salmonella enterica* Typhimurium in meat and meat products using multiplex polymerase chain reaction. *Vet. World* **2017**, *10*, 927–931. [CrossRef] [PubMed]
54. Thong, K.L.; Tan, L.K.; Ooi, P.T. Genetic diversity, virulotyping and antimicrobial resistance susceptibility of *Yersinia enterocolitica* isolated from pigs and porcine products in Malaysia. *J. Sci. Food Agric.* **2017**, *98*, 87–95. [CrossRef]
55. Aguirre, A.A.; Longcore, T.; Barbieri, M.; Dabritz, H.; Hill, D.; Klein, P.N.; Lepczyk, C.; Lilly, E.L.; McLeod, R.; Milcarsky, J.; et al. The One Health Approach to Toxoplasmosis: Epidemiology, Control, and Prevention Strategies. *Ecohealth* **2019**, *16*, 378–390. [CrossRef] [PubMed]
56. Plaza, J.; Dámek, F.; Villena, I.; Innes, E.A.; Katzer, F.; Hamilton, C.M. Detection of *Toxoplasma gondii* in retail meat samples in Scotland. *Food Waterborne Parasitol.* **2020**, *20*, 1–6. [CrossRef] [PubMed]
57. Belluco, S.; Simonato, G.; Mancin, M.; Pietrobelli, M.; Rici, A. *Toxoplasma gondii* infection and food consumption: A systematic review and meta-analysis of case-controlled studies. *Crit. Rev. Food Sci. Nutr.* **2018**, *58*, 3085–3096, . [CrossRef]
58. EFSA. Scientific opinion of the panel on biological hazards on a request from EFSA on surveillance and monitoring of *Toxoplasma* in humans, foods and animals. *EFSA J.* **2007**, *583*, 1–64, . [CrossRef]
59. Van der Giessen, J.; Fonville, M.; Bouwknegt, M.; Langelaar, M.; Vollema, A. Seroprevalence of *Trichinella spiralis* and *Toxoplasma gondii* in pigs from different housing systems in The Netherlands. *Vet. Parasitol.* **2007**, *148*, 371–374. [CrossRef]
60. Opsteegh, M.; Maas, M.; Schares, G.; van der Giessen, J. Relationship between seroprevalence in the main livestock species and presence of *Toxoplasma gondii* in meat (GP/EFSA/BIOHAZ/2013/01) An extensive literature review, Final report. *EFSA Support. Publ.* **2016**, *13*, 1–294. [CrossRef]
61. Gazzonis, A.L.; Marangi, M.; Villa, L.; Ragona, M.E.; Olivieri, E.; Zanzani, S.A.; Giangaspero, A.; Manfredi, M.T. *Toxoplasma gondii* infection and biosecurity levels in fattening pigs and sows: Serological and molecular epidemiology in the intensive pig industry (Lombardy, Northern Italy). *Parasitol. Res.* **2018**, *117*, 539–546, . [CrossRef]
62. Juránková, J.; Basso, W.; Neumayerová, H.; Baláž, V.; Jánová, E.; Sidler, X.; Deplazes, P.; Koudela, B. Brain is the predilection site of *Toxoplasma gondii* in experimentally inoculated pigs as revealed by magnetic capture and real-time PCR. *Food Microbiol.* **2014**, *38*, 167–170, . [CrossRef] [PubMed]
63. Basso, W.; Grimm, F.; Ruetten, M.; Djokić, V.; Blaga, R.; Sidler, X.; Deplazes, P. Experimental *Toxoplasma gondii* infections in pigs: Humoral immune response, estimation of specific IgG avidity and the challenges of reproducing vertical transmission in sows. *Vet. Parasitol.* **2017**, *236*, 76–85, . [CrossRef]
64. Knezić, A.; Zdolec, N. Risk-based meat inspection—The example of the pork chain. *Hrvat. Vet. Vjesn.* **2020**, *28*, 2, 26–32.
65. Franssen, F.; Gerard, C.; Cozma, A.; Vieira-Pinto, M.; Režek Jambrak, A.; Rowan, N.J.; Paulsen, P.; Rozycki, M.; Tysnes, K.; Rodriguez-Lazaro, D.; et al. Inactivation of parasite transmission stages: Efficacy of treatments on food of animal origin. *Trends Food Sci. Technol.* **2019**, *83*, 114–128. [CrossRef]
66. Kijlstra, A.; Jongert, E. Control of the risk of human toxoplasmosis transmitted by meat. *Int. J. Parasitol.* **2008**, *38*, 1359–1370, . [CrossRef]
67. McCurdy, S.M.; Takeuchi, M.T.; Edwards, Z.M.; Edlefsen, M.; Kang, D.H.; Mayes, V.E.; Hillers, V.N. Food safety education initiative to increase consumer use of food thermometers in the United States. *Br. Food J.* **2006**, *108*, 775–794. [CrossRef]
68. Condoleo, R.; Rinaldi, L.; Sette, S.; Mezher, Z. Risk assessment of human toxoplasmosis associated with the consumption of Pork Meat in Italy. *Risk Anal.* **2018**, *38*, 1202–1222, . [CrossRef] [PubMed]
69. Lindsay, D.S.; Collins, M.V.; Holliman, D.; Flick, G.J.; Dubey, J.P. Effects of high-pressure processing on *Toxoplasma gondii* tissue cysts in ground pork. *J. Parasitol.* **2006**, *92*, 195–196. [CrossRef]
70. Opsteegh, M.; Kortbeek, T.M.; Havelaar, A.H.; van Giessen, J.W. Intervention strategies to reduce human *Toxoplasma gondii* disease Burden. *Clin. Infect. Dis.* **2015**, *60*, 101–107. [CrossRef] [PubMed]

71. Pott, S.; Koethe, M.; Bangoura, B.; Zöller, B.; Daugschies, A.; Straubinger, R.K.; Fehlhaber, K.; Ludewig, M. Effects of pH, sodium chloride, and curing salt on the infectivity of *Toxoplasma gondii* tissue cysts. *J. Food Protect.* **2013**, *76*, 1056–1061. [CrossRef]
72. Herrero, L.; Jesús Gracia, M.; Pérez-Arquillué, C.; Lázaro, R.; Herrera, A.; Bayarri, S. *Toxoplasma gondii* in raw and dry-cured ham: The influence of the curing process. *Food Microbiol.* **2017**, *65*, 213–220. [CrossRef] [PubMed]
73. Hill, D.E.; Luchansky, J.; Porto-Fett, A.; Gamble, H.R.; Fournet, V.M.; Hawkins-Cooper, D.S.; Urban, J.F.; Gajadhar, A.A.; Holley, R.; Juneja, V.K.; et al. Rapid inactivation of *Toxoplasma gondii* bradyzoites during formulation of dry cured ready-to-eat pork sausage. *Food Waterborne Parasitol.* **2018**, *12*, 1–7. [CrossRef]

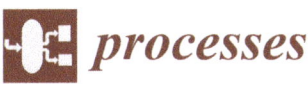

Article

Identification of Microbial Flora in Dry Aged Beef to Evaluate the Rancidity during Dry Aging

Sejeong Kim [1], Jong-Chan Kim [2], Sunhyun Park [2], Jinkwi Kim [2,3], Yohan Yoon [1,4] and Heeyoung Lee [2,*]

[1] Risk Analysis Research Center, Sookmyung Women's University, Seoul 04310, Korea; sjkim_11@naver.com (S.K.); yyoon@sookmyung.ac.kr (Y.Y.)
[2] Food Standard Research Center, Korea Food Research Institute, Wanju 55365, Korea; jckim@kfri.re.kr (J.-C.K.); shpark@kfri.re.kr (S.P.); kimjinkwi@kfri.re.kr (J.K.)
[3] Department of Food Science and Technology, Chung-Ang University, Anseong 17546, Korea
[4] Department of Food and Nutrition, Sookmyung Women's University, Seoul 04310, Korea
* Correspondence: hylee06@kfri.re.kr; Tel.: +82-63-9454

Abstract: Dry aging creates a unique taste and flavor in beef; however, the process also causes rancidity, which is harmful to humans. During dry aging, the microbial flora in beef changes continuously; thus, this change can be used as an indicator of rancidity. The objective of this study was to analyze the correlation between microbial flora in beef and rancidity during dry aging. The round of beef (2.5–3 kg) was dry aged under 1.5 ± 1 °C and $82 \pm 5\%$ moisture for 17 weeks. The microflora in the dry aged beef was analyzed by pyrosequencing. The volatile basic nitrogen (VBN) and thiobarbituric acid reactive substance (TBARS) values were also measured. Primers were designed to detect and quantify bacteria using real-time polymerase chain reaction (RT-PCR). The VBN and TBARS values in the dry aged beef depreciated from week 11 of aging. The levels of *Streptococcus* spp., *Pantoea* spp., and *Pseudomonas* spp. significantly changed at around week 11. Quantitative RT-PCR showed that the levels of *Pantoea* spp. and *Streptococcus* spp. could be used to identify rancidity during dry aging. Thus, among the microbial flora in dry aged beef, *Pantoea* spp. and *Streptococcus* spp. can be used to determine the rancidity of dry aged beef.

Keywords: microbial flora; dry aged beef; rancidity; index

1. Introduction

Dry aging, a process that involves the long-term storage of meat at low temperatures and relative humidity, can improve meat quality, which is represented by the development of tenderness and a unique flavor. These quality factors are considerably affected by aging conditions, such as temperature, air velocity, and humidity [1]. With the increasing interest of consumers in its unique flavor, the dry aged beef market in the United States was expected to reach $11,176 million in 2020 [2]. Dry aged beef is consumed globally, including in Germany, Asia, the Middle East, Europe, and the United States, and the consumption of dry aged beef accounts for <10% of overall beef consumption [3].

In dry aging, during the long-time storage, a tremendous number of microbes are colonized on the surface of the meat (forming "crust"), and the composition of the microbial community keeps changing continuously [4]. Microbes, including bacteria, yeasts, and molds, metabolize ingredients in the meat and produce various metabolites that affect the flavor, tenderness, and rancidity of dry aged meat [5,6]. Therefore, the quality of dry aged beef is related to changes in the microbial community on the meat. For example, *Pseudomonas* spp., the main spoilage bacterium, metabolizes glucose, lactate, and amino acid, which results in the formation of slime and generation of off-odor, while lactic acid bacteria cause greening as a consequence of H_2O_2 generation [7,8]. Psychrotrophs, such as pseudomonads and lactobacilli, largely contribute to the spoilage of meat at chilling temperatures and continuously compete with each other during the storage time.

Under aerobic conditions, *Pseudomonas* species dominate, but lactobacilli dominate under anaerobic conditions by producing an antimicrobial agent that inhibits the growth of other species [9].

Recently, the microbial community on dry aged beef was characterized using metagenomic analysis [4]. In this study, dry aging led to prominent changes in the microbial composition, especially in the abundance of lactic acid bacteria, and some yeast/mold strains were prevalent in dry aged beef for a certain duration. In addition, Lee et al. (2019) [10] revealed the effects of air velocities on changes in microbial composition and on the properties of dry aged beef. Although little is known about the correlation between the microbial community and the quality of dry aged meat, some specific strains, such as *Pilaira anomala* and *Debaryomyces hansenii*, have been proven to have a positive effect on the quality of dry aged meat [10,11]. Based on these findings, it is expected that analysis of the microbial community on dry aged beef can provide information about the quality of the beef.

As the period of dry aging is extended, the quality of the meat gradually decreases. During this period, proteins and lipids are broken down extensively, and meat flavor, tenderness, juiciness, odor, and texture are affected negatively [12]. The rancidity of dry aged beef cannot be easily evaluated based on its appearance. Thiobarbituric acid reactive substance (TBARS) and volatile basic nitrogen (VBN) values are well-known indices for distinguishing the rancidity of meat, because these parameters are quantitative indices of the oxidative deterioration of lipids and ammonia production by deamination of amino acids, respectively [13]. Although some strains, such as *Pseudomonas* spp., and members of Enterobacteriaceae, are known as meat spoilage bacteria [14], the specific microbial strains that can be used to evaluate the rancidity of dry aged beef are not yet known.

Metagenomics is one of the tools for genetic analysis (sequencing and identification), which can be used to study the genetic content of the entire microbial community in certain environments [15]. The analyses start with the extraction of deoxyribonucleic acid (DNA) from the microbial community, and then the genetic information is obtained by random shotgun sequencing, followed by metadata analysis [16]. Given that metagenomics can easily detect anaerobes or newly isolated microorganisms compared with culturing methods [17], metagenomics is widely used for analyzing microflora [18,19]. Therefore, in this study, we aimed to investigate changes in the microbial community during dry aging to find relationships between rancidity and microflora in dry aged beef.

2. Materials and Methods

2.1. Dry Aging of Beef

The round of beef (2.5–3 kg) was purchased from a local market (Seoul, Korea). The whole beef was dry aged in DRY AGER® (DX1000, Landig + Lava GmbH & Co., Bad Saulgau, Germany) at 1.5 ± 1 °C and $82 \pm 5\%$ moisture for 17 weeks. A microbial cluster formed outside of the beef as the aging progressed. A portion (0.25 g) of the cluster (two for each of three samples) was used to analyze the microflora [10] and the microbial level (25 g of the cluster), and the portion of meat inside (10 g) was used to measure the VBN and TBARS values.

2.2. Analysis of Microflora on Beef during Dry Aging

The microbial cluster (0.25 g) that formed outside the beef was collected at certain intervals (1–3 weeks) during dry aging. Microbial DNA was extracted from the cluster using a DNeasy PowerFood Microbial Kit (Cat. No. 21000-100; Qiagen, Hilden, Germany) according to the manufacturer's instructions. Briefly, the cluster samples in 2 mL microcentrifuge tubes were homogenized with MBL buffer (a cell lysis buffer) using a Vortex Adapter (Cat. No. 13000-V1-24; Qiagen, Hilden, Germany) and vortexed thoroughly. After centrifuging the lysate at $13,000 \times g$ for 1 min, an IRS solution (inhibitor removal solution) was added to the supernatant, and the mixture was refrigerated at 4 °C for 5 min to remove contaminants. Centrifugation was repeated, and the supernatants were transferred to a new 2 mL collection tube. To induce the DNA to bind the membrane in the column, the supernatants were mixed with solution MR (highly concentrated salt solution), and the mixtures were loaded onto the MB spin columns and centrifuged. After washing, the DNA was eluted with 100 µL of solution EB (elution buffer). The DNA samples were subjected to meta-analysis using an Illumina MiSeq Sequencing system (SY-410-1003, Illumina, San Diego, CA, USA), and the sequencing data were then clustered using Cluster Database at High Identity with Tolerance (CD-HIT) and UCLUST. Processing of raw reads started with quality check, and filtering of low quality (<Q25) reads using Trimmomatic ver. 0.32. After QC-pass results, paired-end sequence data were merged using the fastq_mergepairs command of VSEARCH version 2.13.4 with default parameters. Primers were then trimmed with the alignment algorithm of Myers and Miller at a similarity cut-off of 0.8. Non-specific amplicons that do not encode 16S rRNA were detected by nhmmer in HMMER software package ver. 3.2.1 with hmm profiles. Principal coordinates analysis (PCoA), which converts data on distances between items into a map-based visualization, was conducted using EzBioCloud Program (Chunlab, Inc., Seoul, Korea).

2.3. Quantitative Polymerase Chain Reaction PCR (q-PCR)

The bacterial on the dry aged beef (25 g) were quantified using q-PCR. The primer sequences used in this study are listed in Table 1. A primer targeting *Pantoea* spp. was developed in this study, and its sensitivity and specificity were verified using various bacterial strains, such as *Pseudomonas* spp. and *Streptococcus* spp. (Supplementary Table S1; Supplementary Figure S1). For q-PCR, the reaction mixture was prepared in a 0.1 mL Strip q-PCR tube (Cat. No. 981103; Qiagen, Hilden, Germany) as follows: 12.5 µL of 2× Rotor-Gene SYBR Green PCR Master Mix (Cat. No. 204074; Qiagen, Hilden, Germany), 2.5 µL of primer_foward (10 µM), 2.5 µL of primer_reverse (10 µM), 6.5 µL of ribonuclease (RNase)-free water, and 1 µL of DNA template. The mixture was amplified using Rotor-GeneQ (Qiagen) at 95 °C for 5–35 cycles (95 °C, 5–60 °C, 10 s). The cycle threshold (C_t) value was converted to the bacterial level using the standard curve of each primer (Supplementary Figure S2).

Table 1. Primers used to detect bacteria on dry aged beef.

Strain	Primer (3'–5')	Target Gene	Reference
Pantoea spp.	F: CACTGGAAACGGTGGCTAAT R: CTGGGTTCATCCGATAGTGAG	16S rRNA	This study
Pseudomonas spp.	F: ACTTTAAGTTGGGAGGAAGGG R: ACACAGGAAATTCCACCACCC	16S rRNA	[20]
Streptococcus spp.	F: CGATACATAGCCGACCTGAGA R: CCACTCTCCCCTYYTGCAC	16S rRNA	[21]
Universal bacteria			
Gram-positive	F: GAAAGTCCGGGCTCCATA R: ATAAGCCGGGTTCTGT	mp(G−)	[22]
Gram-negative	F: GAGGAAATCCRKGCTCGCAC R: AGGGGTTTACCGCGTTCC	mp(G+)	[22]

rRNA, ribosomal ribonucleic acid.

2.4. Measurement of the TBARS and VBN Values

The TBARS values were determined according to the method of Witte et al. (1970) [23] with slight modifications. Briefly, beef samples (10 g) were blended for 1 min in a homogenizer (CH580, Hai Xin Technology Company, Shenzhen, China) with water three times the amount of the sample. The homogenate was filtered through an Advantec No. 1 filter paper (Cat. No. 265172; Chiba, Japan), and the filtrate was mixed with 20 mM 2-thiobarbituric acid and 20% trichloroacetic acid. The mixtures were reacted at 99 °C in a water bath, and the reaction was stopped by cooling under running water. After filtration, the absorbance of the samples at 531 nm was measured using a spectrophotometer (BioTek Instruments, Winooski, VT, USA). The VBN value was measured using microdiffusion analysis [24]. The beef sample (10 g) was homogenized in distilled water to a volume of 100 mL using a mess flask. The homogenate was filtered through a filter paper. One milliliter of the filtrate was transferred to the outer part of a Conway dish, and then 1 mL of 0.01 N boric acid (H_3BO_3) and 0.1 mL of Conway solution (0.066% methyl red + 0.066% bromocresol green in ethanol) was transferred to the inner part. A 50% potassium carbonate (K_2CO_3) solution was added to the lower layer of the outer part. The dish was then sealed and incubated at 37 °C for 2 h. Finally, a drop of 0.02 N sulfuric acid (H_2SO_4) was added to the inner part until the color changed from green to red, and the VBN value was calculated.

2.5. Statistical Analysis

The experiment was replicated with three samples. Data for the microflora were analyzed using the Wilcoxon rank-sum test. Data for the level of quality factors (TBARS, VBN, and bacterial level) in dry aged beef were analyzed using Analysis of Variance (ANOVA) with SPSS statistical software (SPSS Ver. 20.0; IBM, Chicago, IL, USA). Least square means among the groups were compared using a Tukey's range test at $\alpha = 0.05$.

3. Results and Discussion

3.1. Changes in the Level of Quality Factors during Dry Aging of Beef

Lipid oxidation and protein putrefaction are highly related to a decrease in taste and flavor in spoiled meat, which are reflected in the TBARS and VBN values, respectively. At low temperatures, the pH of meat is increased as the meat is spoiled, and this causes an increase in the water-holding capacity of the meat [25]. In this study, round beef was dry aged under low temperature for a long time, and its quality factors, including TBARS, VBN, and water holding capacity (WHC), were analyzed at certain intervals during 24 weeks of dry aging. The TBARS value was significantly increased at the fifth week, and the VBN value increased at the 14th week of dry aging ($p < 0.05$) (Figure 1A,B). The WHC of beef considerably increased after the 11th week ($p < 0.05$) (Figure 1C). These results indicate that the quality of dry aged beef decreased from the 11th week. Therefore, the dry aging duration was divided into early and late stages based on the 11th week, the time at which the quality of the dry aged beef decreased.

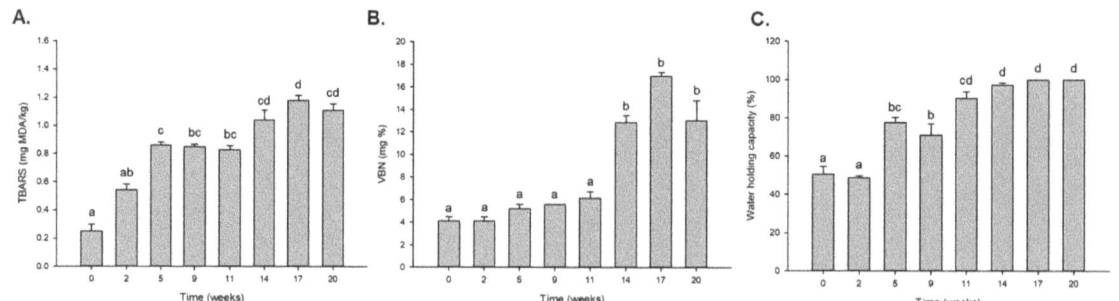

Figure 1. Changes in the (**A**) thiobarbituric acid reactive substance (TBARS), (**B**) volatile basic nitrogen (VBN), and (**C**) water holding capacity values in the dry aged beef during an aging time of 24 weeks. a–d: means with different letters are significantly different ($p < 0.05$). The data were analyzed using Analysis of Variance (ANOVA).

3.2. Changes in the Composition of Microflora during Dry Aging of Beef

The microflora that colonized on the surface of the dry aged beef (cluster) were analyzed using metagenomics analysis at 0–24 weeks of age. The number of valid reads ranged from 14,817 to 115,681. PCoA showed that the composition of microflora was grouped by dry aging duration (Supplementary Figure S3). To facilitate the analysis, the data were divided into two groups: early (~11th week) and late (~11th week), and the compositions of the two groups were compared. Diversity indices of microflora, such as Chao1, abundance-based coverage estimator (ACE), and Jackknife, were significantly lower in the early group than in the late group ($p < 0.05$) (Figure 2A). This result indicates that the diversity of the microflora is correlated with the rancidity of dry aged beef. Similar results were observed in a previous study [24]. In the previous study, differences between fresh and low-temperature spoiled round beef were compared, and it was observed that the general type of flora changed from mixed and many types of microflora in the fresh meat to homogeneous and few types of microflora in the spoiled meat. Similar trends of decreased microbial diversity in spoiled meats were observed in other types of red meats and under various storage conditions [26,27].

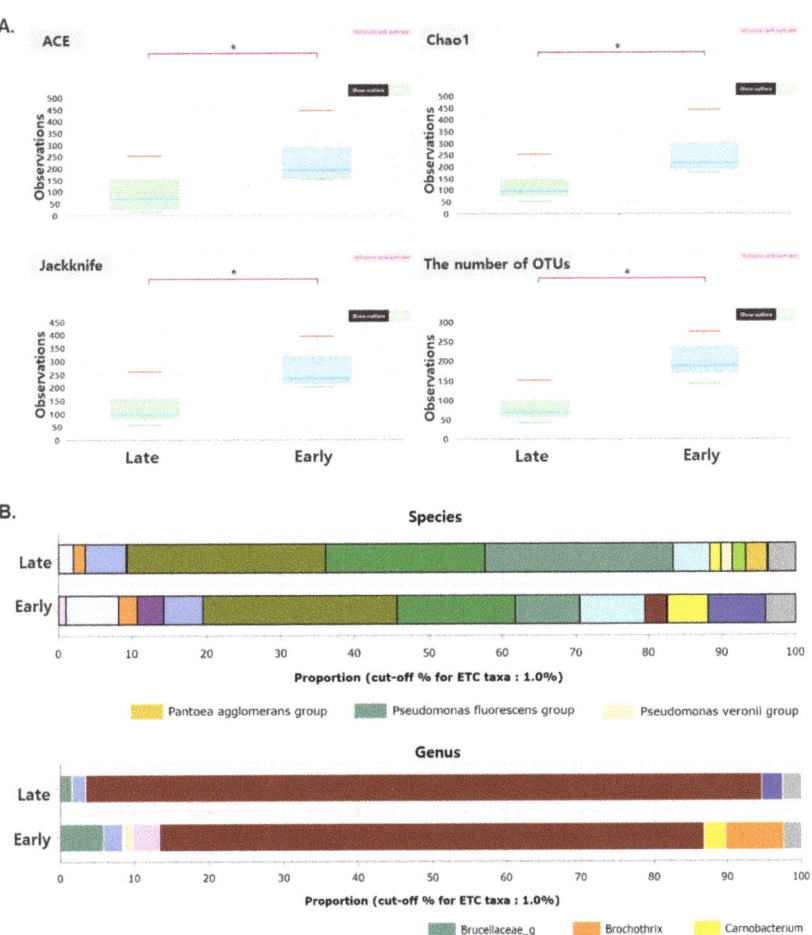

Figure 2. Metagenomic analysis of the microflora in the early (before the 11th week) or late stage (after the 11th week) of dry aging. (**A**) Diversity indices; and (**B**) microbial composition at the genus and species levels. * indicates that the two groups are significantly different ($p < 0.05$). The data were analyzed using Wilcoxon rank-sum test.

The microflora was further analyzed to investigate the microbial strains and determine the rancidity of the dry aged beef. At the species level, the compositions of the *Pantoea agglomerans*, *Pseudomonas fluorescens*, and *Pseudomonas veronii* groups were higher in the late group than in the early group (Figure 2B). At the genus level, the composition of microorganisms, such as Brucellaceae, *Brochothrix*, and *Carnobacterium*, was higher in the early group compared with that in the late group (Figure 2B). These differences in the microbial composition between the early and late groups mean that the dry aging process (also decrease in quality) is highly correlated with the composition of the microbial community. However, the specific relationship between the quality and the microbial community of dry aged beef has hitherto not been clearly understood.

In particular, the relative abundances of *Pantoea* spp. and *Pseudomonas* spp. were significantly higher in the late group than in the early group, while that of *Streptococcus* spp. was significantly lower in the late group ($p < 0.05$) (Figure 3). Similar changes in relative bacterial levels of *Pseudomonas* spp. and *Streptococcus* spp. have been observed in previous studies [4,28]. *Pantoea*, a genus belonging to the Enterobacteriaceae family, contributes to meat spoilage [29]. *Pseudomonas* spp. are well-known psychrotrophic bacteria, which are often isolated from spoiled meat, and *Pseudomonas fragi*, *Pseudomonas lundensis*, and *Pseudomonas fluorescens* are frequently found species [5]. *Streptococcus* is a genus of lactic acid bacteria, which are the most abundant strains in the early stage of dry aging, but their number decreases as ripening progresses [4]. These genera are commonly found in meat that is spoiled/stored in air [5]. Therefore, together with the results from Figure 1, changes in the abundance of *Pantoea* spp., *Pseudomonas* spp., and *Streptococcus* spp. could be used to determine the rancidity of dry aged beef.

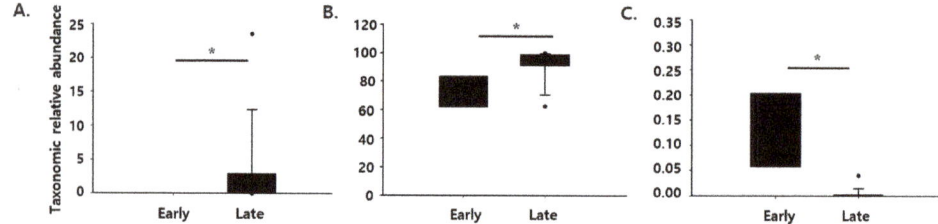

Figure 3. Bacterial levels in the early (before the 11th week) or late stage (after the 11th week) of dry aging observed using the 16S sequencing-based method. (**A**) *Pantoea* spp., (**B**) *Pseudomonas* spp., and (**C**) *Streptococcus* spp. * indicates that the two groups are significantly different ($p < 0.05$). The data were analyzed using Wilcoxon rank-sum test.

3.3. Level of the Microbes Quantified Using Real-Time q-PCR (qRT-PCR) during Dry Aging in Beef

To validate the use of *Pantoea* spp., *Pseudomonas* spp., and *Streptococcus* spp. as indices for the rancidity of dry aged beef, the abundance of these microbes was quantified in newly produced dry aged beef using qRT-PCR. In the initial stage, the number of *Pantoea* spp. was 3.7 log CFU/g, which increased during the early stage of dry aging (Figure 2). The number of *Pantoea* spp. was significantly decreased after the 10th week of dry aging ($p < 0.05$), and it was 2.3 log CFU/g at the very late stage of dry aging (the 17th week). This result indicates that the number of *Pantoea* spp. is highly related to the quality of dry aged beef. Li et al. (2020) [30] also found that the number of *Pantoea* spp. was lower in spoiled meat products compared with that in normal meat products. However, these results are different from that of the microflora analysis in the present study, which showed a decreased abundance of *Pantoea* spp. in the late group (Figure 3). The reason for these differences could be as follows: (1) differences between "composition" in the microflora analysis and "quantity" in the qRT-PCR analysis; and/or (2) limitation of primers that could cover all strains of *Pantoea* spp. on the beef.

The number of *Pseudomonas* spp. increased initially and slightly decreased, but not significantly, in the late stage of dry aging (Figure 4). It was also reported in a previous study that *Pseudomonas* spp. (most are *P. fragi*, *P. flourescens*, and *P. lundensis*) were prevalent both in the fresh and spoiled meat [7,25]. Increase in *Pseudomonas* spp. composition in the microflora analysis might be due to a decrease in the total number of microorganisms. This result indicates that *Pseudomonas* spp. cannot be used to determine the rancidity of dry aged beef. Similar results were observed for *Streptococcus* spp. The number of strains gradually decreased after the sixth week of dry aging, but it was not significant (Figure 4). At the 17th week of dry aging, however, the number of *Streptococcus* spp. was significantly decreased to 1.4 log CFU/g. The results indicate that the abundance of *Streptococcus* spp. can be used to determine rancidity in the very late stage of dry aging of beef.

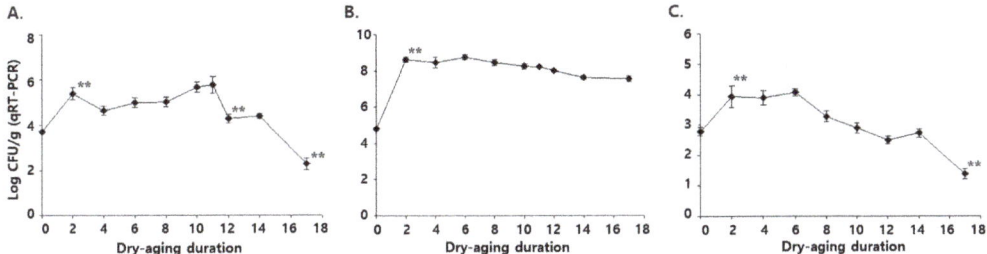

Figure 4. Levels of (**A**) *Pantoea* spp., (**B**) *Pseudomonas* spp., and (**C**) *Streptococcus* spp. measured using qRT-PCR during dry aging of beef. ** indicates that the points are significantly different from those in the previous week ($p < 0.05$). The data were analyzed using Analysis of Variance (ANOVA).

4. Conclusions

In this study, changes in the microbial community during dry aging were investigated, and it was proven that microbial strains are highly related to the rancidity of dry aged beef. Based on the microflora analysis and quantification using qRT-PCR, *Pantoea* spp. and *Streptococcus* spp. could be used to determine the rancidity of dry aged beef. Findings from this study might be helpful for manufacturers to manage the decay of dry aged beef. Further studies are needed to validate the use of these strains under various conditions of dry aging or in applications with other parts of beef.

Supplementary Materials: The following are available online at https://www.mdpi.com/article/10.3390/pr9112049/s1, Figure S1: Sensitivity and specificity of primers used to detect *Pantoea* spp.; Figure S2: Standard curve for each primer used to detect bacteria in the study; Figure S3: Metagenomic analysis on the microflora on the dry aged beef (0–20 weeks). (a) Principal coordinates analysis (PoCA) graph; (b) diversity indices; and (c) microbial composition at the species level; Table S1: Bacterial strains used in this study.

Author Contributions: Conceptualization, S.K., Y.Y. and H.L.; methodology, S.K.; formal analysis, S.K., S.P. and J.K.; investigation, S.K., S.P., J.K. and H.L.; data curation, S.K. and H.L.; writing—original draft preparation, S.K.; writing—review and editing, J.-C.K., Y.Y. and H.L.; supervision, J.-C.K.; project administration, J.-C.K. All authors have read and agreed to the published version of the manuscript.

Funding: This research was supported by the Main Research Program (E0211400-01) of the Korea Food Research Institute (KFRI), funded by the Ministry of Science and ICT (Korea).

Conflicts of Interest: The authors declare no conflict of interest.

References

1. Kim, Y.H.B.; Kemp, R.; Samuelsson, L.M. Effects of dry-aging on meat quality attributes and metabolite profiles of beef Loins. *Meat Sci.* **2016**, *111*, 168–176. [CrossRef]
2. Allied Market Research. U.S. Dry Aging Beef Market–Opportunity Analysis and Industry Forecast, 2014–2020. Available online: https://www.alliedmarketresearch.com/US-dry-aging-beef-market (accessed on 5 November 2021).
3. Ashaman, H.; Hastie, M.; Warner, R.; Jacob, R.; Hunyh, L. Dry-Aging—Introduction and Insights. Available online: https://www.mla.com.au/globalassets/mla-corporate/news-and-events/documents/dry-ageing-meat/introduction-and-market-insights (accessed on 5 November 2021).
4. Ryu, S.; Shin, M.; Cho, S.; Hwang, I.; Kim, Y.; Oh, S. Microbial and fungal communities on dry aged beef of Hanwoo using metagenomic analysis. *Foods* **2020**, *9*, 1571. [CrossRef] [PubMed]

5. Casaburi, A.; Piombino, P.; Nychas, G.J.; Villani, F.; Ercolini, D. Bacterial populations and the volatilome associated to meat spoilage. *Food Microbiol.* **2015**, *45*, 83–102. [CrossRef]
6. Terkimg, N.; Witte, F.; Heinz, V. The dry aged beef paradox: Why dry aging is sometimes not better than wet aging. *Meat Sci.* **2021**, *172*, 108355.
7. Raposo, A.; Perez, E.; de Faria, C.T.; Ferrus, M.A.; Carrascosa, C. Chapter 3—Food Spoilage by *Pseudomonas* spp. An Overview. In *Foodborne Pathogens and Antibiotic Resistance*; Singh, O.V., Ed.; John Wiley & Sons, Inc.: Hoboken, NJ, USA, 2016; pp. 21–39.
8. Nychas, G.-J.E.; Marshall, D.; Sofos, J. Chapter 6—Meat Poultry and Seafood; In *Food Microbiology Fundamentals and Frontiers*; Doyle, M.P., Beuchat, L.R., Montville, T.J., Eds.; ASM Press: New York, NY, USA, 2007.
9. Gill, C.O.; Newton, K.G. The ecology of bacterial spoilage of fresh meat at chill temperatures. *Meat Sci.* **1978**, *2*, 207–217. [CrossRef]
10. Lee, H.J.; Yoon, J.W.; Kim, M.; Oh, H.; Yoon, Y.; Jo, C. Changes in microbial composition on the crust by different air flow velocities and their effect on sensory properties of dry aged beef. *Meat Sci.* **2019**, *153*, 152–158. [CrossRef] [PubMed]
11. Oh, H.; Lee, H.J.; Lee, J.; Jo, C.; Yoon, Y. Identification of microorganisms associated with the quality improvement of dry aged beef through microbiome analysis and DNA sequencing, and evaluation of their effects on beef quality. *J. Food Sci.* **2019**, *84*, 2944–2954. [CrossRef] [PubMed]
12. Dave, D.; Ghaly, A.E. Meat spoilage mechanisms and preservation techniques: A critical review. *Am. J. Agric. Biol. Sci.* **2011**, *6*, 486–510.
13. Byun, J.S.; Min, J.S.; Kim, I.S.; Chung, M.S.; Lee, M. Comparison of indicators of microbial quality of meat during aerobic cold storage. *J. Food Prot.* **2003**, *66*, 1733–1737. [CrossRef]
14. Borch, E.; Kant-Muermans, M.L.; Blixt, Y. Bacterial spoilage of meat and cured meat products. *Int. J. Food Microbiol.* **1996**, *33*, 103–120. [CrossRef]
15. Govindarajulu, S.N.; Varier, K.M.; Jayamurali, D.; Liu, W.; Chen, J.; Manoharan, N.; Li, Y.; Gajendran, B. Chapter 16—Insect Gut Microbiome and Its Applications. In *Recent Advancements in Microbial Diversity*; De Mandal, S., Bhatt, P., Eds.; Academic Press: Cambridge, MA, USA, 2020; pp. 379–395.
16. Thomas, T.; Gilbert, J.; Meyer, F. Metagenomics—A guide from sampling to data analysis. *Microb. Inform. Exp.* **2012**, *2*, 3. [CrossRef]
17. Neelakanta, G.; Sultana, H. The use of metagenomic approaches to analyze changes in microbial communities. *Microbiol. Insights* **2013**, *6*, 37–48. [CrossRef] [PubMed]
18. Yang, S.; Gao, X.; Meng, J.; Zhang, A.; Zhou, Y.; Long, M.; Li, B.; Deng, W.; Jin, L.; Zhao, S.; et al. Metagenomic analysis of bacteria, fungi, bacteriophages, and helminths in the gut of giant pandas. *Front. Microbiol.* **2018**, *9*, 1717. [CrossRef]
19. Wang, W.; Xu, S.; Ren, Z.; Tao, L.; Jiang, J.; Zheng, S. Application of metagenomics in the human gut microbiome. *World J. Gastroenterol.* **2015**, *21*, 803–814. [CrossRef] [PubMed]
20. Bergmark, L.; Poulsen, P.H.B.; Al-Soud, W.A.; Norman, A.; Hansen, L.H.; Sørensen, S.J. Assessment of the specificity of *Burkholderia* and *Pseudomonas* qPCR assays for detection of these genera in soil using 454 pyrosequencing. *FEMS Microbiol. Lett.* **2012**, *333*, 77–84. [CrossRef]
21. Chumponsuk, T.; Jaroensuk, S.; Phengkhot, S.; Gentekaki, E.; Popluechai, S.; Kullawong, N. Development of genus-specific primers for quantitative PCR analysis of *Streptococcus* in human feces. In Proceeding of the 29th Annual Meeting of the Thai Society for Biotechnology and International Conference, Bangkok, Thailand, 23–25 November 2017.
22. Dolan, A.; Burgess, C.M.; Barry, T.B.; Fanning, S.; Duffy, G. A novel quantitative reverse-transcription PCR (qRT-PCR) for the enumeration of total bacteria, using meat micro-flora as a model. *J. Microbiol. Methods* **2009**, *77*, 1–7. [CrossRef] [PubMed]
23. Witte, V.C.; Krause, G.F.; Bailey, M.E. A new extraction method for determining 2-thiobarbituric acid values of pork and beef during storage. *J. Food Sci.* **1970**, *35*, 582–585. [CrossRef]
24. Conway, E.J.; Byrne, A. An absorption apparatus for the micro-determination of certain volatile substances: The micro-determination of ammonia. *Biochem. J.* **1933**, *27*, 419–429.
25. Jay, J.M. Mechanism and detection of microbial spoilage in meats at low temperatures: A status report. *J. Milk Food Technol.* **1972**, *35*, 467–471. [CrossRef]
26. Li, M.Y.; Zhou, G.H.; Xu, X.L.; Li, C.B.; Zhu, W.Y. Changes of bacterial diversity and main flora in chilled pork during storage using PCR-DGGE. *Food Micobiol.* **2006**, *23*, 607–611. [CrossRef] [PubMed]
27. Dainty, R.H.; Mackey, B.M. The relationship between the phenotypic properties of bacteria from chill-stored meat and spoilage processes. *J. Appl. Microbiol.* **1992**, *73*, 103S–114S. [CrossRef] [PubMed]
28. Ercolini, D.; Russo, F.; Torrieri, E.; Masi, P.; Villani, F. Changes in the spoilage-related microbiota of beef during refrigerated storage under different packaging conditions. *Appl. Environ. Microbiol.* **2006**, *72*, 4663–4671. [CrossRef] [PubMed]
29. Li, R.; Cai, L.; Gao, T.; Li, C.; Zhou, G.; Ye, K. Comparing the quality characteristics and bacterial communities in meatballs with or without blown pack spoilage. *LWT* **2020**, *130*, 109529. [CrossRef]
30. Oh, H.; Kim, S.; Lee, S.; Lee, H.; Ha, J.; Lee, J.; Choi, Y.; Choi, K.H.; Yoon, Y. Prevalence, serotype diversity, genotype and antibiotic resistance of *Listeria monocytogenes* isolated from carcasses and human in Korea. *Food Sci. Anim. Resour.* **2018**, *38*, 851–865. [CrossRef]

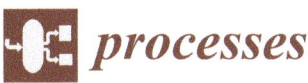

Article

The Influence of Surface Mycobiota on Sensory Properties of "Istarski pršut" and "Dalmatinski pršut"

Tina Lešić [1], Nada Vahčić [2], Ivica Kos [3], Manuela Zadravec [4], Dragan Milićević [5], Irena Perković [6], Eddy Listeš [7] and Jelka Pleadin [1,*]

[1] Laboratory for Analytical Chemistry, Croatian Veterinary Institute, Savska Cesta 143, 10000 Zagreb, Croatia; lesic@veinst.hr
[2] Faculty of Food Technology and Biotechnology, University of Zagreb, Pierottijeva 6, 10000 Zagreb, Croatia; nvahcic@pbf.hr
[3] Department of Animal Science and Technology, Faculty of Agriculture, University of Zagreb, Svetošimunska Cesta 25, 10000 Zagreb, Croatia; ikos@agr.hr
[4] Laboratory for Feed Microbiology, Croatian Veterinary Institute, Savska Cesta 143, 10000 Zagreb, Croatia; zadravec@veinst.hr
[5] Institute of Meat Hygiene and Technology, Kaćanskog 13, 11040 Belgrade, Serbia; dragan.milicevic@inmes.rs
[6] Regional Veterinary Institute Vinkovci, Croatian Veterinary Institute, Ul. Josipa Kozarca 24, 32100 Vinkovci, Croatia; perkovicirena1512@gmail.com
[7] Regional Veterinary Institute Split, Croatian Veterinary Institute, Poljička Cesta 33, 21000 Split, Croatia; e.listes.vzs@veinst.hr
* Correspondence: pleadin@veinst.hr

Citation: Lešić, T.; Vahčić, N.; Kos, I.; Zadravec, M.; Milićević, D.; Perković, I.; Listeš, E.; Pleadin, J. The Influence of Surface Mycobiota on Sensory Properties of "Istarski pršut" and "Dalmatinski pršut". *Processes* 2021, 9, 2287. https://doi.org/10.3390/pr9122287

Received: 2 December 2021
Accepted: 17 December 2021
Published: 20 December 2021

Publisher's Note: MDPI stays neutral with regard to jurisdictional claims in published maps and institutional affiliations.

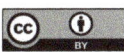

Copyright: © 2021 by the authors. Licensee MDPI, Basel, Switzerland. This article is an open access article distributed under the terms and conditions of the Creative Commons Attribution (CC BY) license (https://creativecommons.org/licenses/by/4.0/).

Abstract: This study aimed to identify surface mould species overgrowing the Croatian protected meat products "Istarski pršut" and "Dalmatinski pršut" and their effect on sensory properties. Dry-cured hams were produced in 2018/2019 and obtained from annual fairs. The predominant surface species found on "Dalmatinski pršut" were *Aspergillus chevalieri*, *Penicillium citrinum* and *Aspergillus cibarius*, whereas those overgrowing "Istarski pršut" were *Aspergillus proliferans*, *P. citrinum* and *Penicillium salamii*. The results show species diversity, higher presence, and greater variety of *Aspergillus* species in "Dalmatinski pršut" in comparison to "Istarski pršut", and significant variations in 9 of 20 sensory attributes. Principal component analysis revealed a clear distinction between the two, and a large contribution of *P. salamii* and *Penicillium bialowienzense* to one principal component. The texture traits, smoky odour, muscle and subcutaneous fatty tissue colour, and mould species found are valuable for product characterisation. The results also indicate that mould species may be responsible for some sensory traits, such as tenderness, juiciness, and lesser freshness.

Keywords: meat products; dry-cured hams; sensory evaluation; surface moulds; *Penicillium*; *Aspergillus*; Croatian regions

1. Introduction

The production of dry-cured hams is traditionally associated with European Mediterranean countries, especially Spain, Italy, France, and Croatia, as the countries of origin of numerous different ham types [1–4]. These products are recognised and highly prized for their delicious odour, flavour, and texture [3]. A dry-cured ham is a cured meat product whose preparation involves dry salting, dehydration, and gradual chemical-enzymatic transformations of fresh pork during long-term ripening (over 12 months). These basic production components are common to all types of dry-cured hams, but it should be emphasised that raw material and some technological and environmental production aspects can differ significantly, resulting in different sensory properties of the final product [4]. The most famous Croatian dry-cured hams are Protected Geographical Indication (PGI)-labelled "Dalmatinski pršut" and Protected Designation of Origin (PDO)-labelled "Istarski pršut" [5,6], both belonging to the EU geographical indication schemes that protect products coming from a specific region in which traditional production takes place. Regarding the PDO-labelled products, raw ingredients come from the region of origin where the entire production takes place, whereas in the case of the PGIs, at least one of the production stages takes place in the region.

Sensory quality of dry-cured meat products depends on various factors, such as the quality of meat raw materials and other ingredients, processing conditions, and microbial ecology. Microbiota involved in ripening and fermentation processes are diverse and complex, and comprise bacteria, yeasts, and moulds [7]. Moulds overgrow the surface of these products during the production process and are characteristic of the production area [8]. Moulds overgrow prosciuttos within a month and a half, and gradually colonise their entire surface [9]. Surface mould abundance and their subsequent spiderweb-like residua are one of the distinctive characteristics of "Istarski pršut" and an indicator of its proper drying and ripening [5]. The predominant mould genera isolated from the surface of these products are *Penicillium* and *Aspergillus* [9–12], because dry-cured meat products are mostly composed of water, proteins and lipids, and therefore represent a rich substrate that can enhance mould growth. At the same time, however, high salt content, low a_w and low ripening temperatures make the surface of these products almost mould-unfriendly. However, these genera are well-adapted to these xerophilic and halophilic conditions and therefore capable of dominating throughout the ripening period [4,12,13].

Surface mould present on these products is generally appreciated because of its enzymatic activity, such as lipolysis, lipid oxidation, proteolysis, and amino acid degradation, which contribute to the development of a characteristic dry-cured ham flavour. Lipolysis is the first step to free fatty acids' oxidation. Secondary fatty acid reactions result in numerous oxidation products, such as aldehydes, alcohols, ketones and others [8,14,15]. Moulds also contain enzymes that can hydrolyse muscle proteins, contributing to the proteolysis and the release of amino acids [8,16]. The presence of surface moulds on dry-cured meat products has other desirable effects, such as the establishment of surface microclimate able to prevent crust formation and flavour diminishment, in addition to antioxidant activity due to oxygen consumption, and a mycelium barrier effect that reduces the penetration of oxygen and light, thus preserving the colour and taste of the product and delaying its rancidity. Surface moulds can also be protective against pathogenic microorganisms [13,17–19]. Nonetheless, if mould growth is not controlled during the production process, unwanted species can be developed, which can affect the sensory properties of the products and reduce their quality through antibiotic and mycotoxin contamination responsible for consumer allergic reactions, antibiotic resistance, and acute and chronic toxicity [13,20].

Dry-cured hams traditionally produced in households are usually not inoculated with starter cultures and are often produced under relatively uncontrolled conditions. As a result, depending on the production area, uncontrolled moulds can appear on their surface and affect different sensory properties [8]. The main differences between "Dalmatinski pršut" and "Istarski pršut" are the geographical region of origin and some technological aspects of their production, because "Istarski pršut", as opposed to "Dalmatinski pršut", is skinless and unsmoked [5,6]. Although some research on the contribution of certain mould species to lipolysis, proteolysis and volatile compounds of dry-cured meat products has been undertaken, the contribution of fungal population to flavour formation and the role of fungi in big meat pieces, such as dry-cured hams, remain unclear. Of note, regarding dry-cured meat products, the most extensively studied mould species are those that can be used as starter cultures such as *P. nalgiovense*, *P. chrysogenum* and *P. camemberti*, whereas the contribution of other species to sensory properties of these products has been poorly investigated [8,14,16–18,21].

Several studies of sensory properties of Croatian protected products "Istarski pršut" and "Dalmatinski pršut", considered to be among the most important traditional dry-cured meat products produced in different Croatian regions, have been conducted in relation to volatile compounds [4,15,22–24]. However, to the best of our knowledge, to date only one study identified surface moulds overgrowing these long-ripened dry-cured meat products [12], and the relationship between surface moulds and the sensory properties of these products has not been studied yet. This study aimed to identify surface mould species overgrowing "Dalmatinski pršut" and "Istarski pršut" and the effect of surface mycobiota on the sensory properties of the final products.

2. Materials and Methods

2.1. Dry-Cured Ham Production and Sampling

For the purposes of this study, samples of "Istarski pršut" ($n = 15$) and "Dalmatinski pršut" ($n = 20$) were retrieved from annual fairs held in Istria (west Croatia) and Dalmatia (south Croatia) during 2019. Samples were taken in the amount of 1.5 to 2 kg and were cut of the caudal part of each ham containing m. semimembranosus, m. semitendinosus and m. biceps femoris.

Dry-cured hams were produced in 2018/2019 using traditional recipes and starter culture-free technologies by different producers located in the two regions according to [4,24,25] with slight modifications. Traditional production is characterised by semi-controlled production conditions, so that differences between manufacturers are possible, but major deviations from product specifications are neither allowed nor were found, given that these meat products are marketed as the products of the Protected Designation of Origin ("Istarski pršut") or the Protected Geographical Indication ("Dalmatinski pršut"). "Dalmatinski pršut" samples were trimmed off without pelvic bones, but with skin and subcutaneous adipose tissue, and "Istarski pršut" samples were trimmed off with pelvic bones, but without skin and subcutaneous adipose tissue. Regarding "Dalmatinski pršut", dry salting made use of coarse and table sea salt, whereas "Istarski pršut" was salted using a combination of coarse and table sea salt supplemented with spices (ground black pepper, laurel and rosemary). On the occasion of the first salting, a total of 30 to 40 g of salt per kg of ham was added, and at the second salting 20 to 30 g of salt per kg was added. The salting took place in cooling chambers at a temperature of 0–5 °C and relative humidity of 80–90% for up to a month, depending on the raw ham weight. After the salting phase, the pressing of hams using approximately 0.1 kg cm^{-2} was applied for 7 days. Drying of both ham types took place in chambers with controlled microclimatic conditions (temperature 12–16 °C; relative humidity 85 to 70%). At the beginning of the "Dalmatinski pršut" drying phase, cold smoke was applied for 20 days at temperatures lower than 22 °C. After 4 months of drying, the hams were moved into ripening chambers operating at the temperatures of 13–18 °C and relative humidity of 65–75%. The production of "Dalmatinski pršut" takes 15 months, and the production of "Istarski pršut" takes 17 months.

2.2. Isolation and Traditional Identification of Surface Mycobiota

Immediately after dry-cured hams' delivery, visible mould colonies were removed from (cut off) the surface using a scalpel, followed by the swabbing of the entire sample surface using damp swabs, with particular attention thereby being paid to the slots (unevenness) present on it. The samples were subsequently transferred onto a DG-18 agar (dichloran 18%-glycerol, Merck, Darmstadt, Germany). After a seven-day incubation in darkness at 25 ± 1 °C, individual mould cultures were sub-cultivated on DG-18 agar, malt extract agar (MEA, BD Difco, Franklin Lakes, NY, USA) and Czapek yeast extract agar (CYA, BD Difco, Franklin Lakes, NY, USA) and incubated for seven days at 25 ± 1 °C in darkness to the end of identification using a traditional method based on macro- and micro-morphology and growth characteristics according to [26,27].

2.3. Molecular Identification of Surface Mycobiota

The outcome of the traditional mould identification was corroborated using a molecular method. DNA was first extracted from isolated mould colonies using a DNeasy Plant Mini Kit (Qiagen, Hilden, Germany) according to the manufacturer's instructions. Primers specific for beta-tubulin (benA)—The Bt2a forward primer (5′-GGTAACCAAATCGGTGCT

GCTTTC-3′) and the Bt2b reverse primer (5′-ACCCTCAGTGTAGTGACCCTTGGC-3′)—and calmodulin (CaM) loci—the Cmd5 forward primer (5′-CCGAGTACAAGGARGCCTTC-3′) and the Cmd6 reverse primer (5′-CCGATRGAGGTCATRACGTGG-3′)—were selected for polymerase chain reaction (PCR) amplification (Macrogen, Amsterdam, The Netherlands). The reaction mixture (25 µL) was prepared using 1 µL of the template DNA, 12.5 µL of 2× PCR buffer (HotStarTaq Plus MasterMix Kit, Qiagen, Hilden, Germany), 2.5 µL of 10× Coral Load, 0.4 µM of each primer, and nuclease-free water. PCR was performed in a 51149-2 thermal cycler (Prime Thermal Cycler, Staffordshire, UK) under the following cycling conditions: 95 °C for 5 min followed by 40 cycles at 94 °C for 30 s, 56 °C for 30 s, 72 °C for 60 s, concluding with 72 °C for 10 min. PCR products were checked using gel electrophoresis in 1.5%-agarose gel and visualised using UV trans-illumination (UVIDOC, UVITEC, Cambridge, UK). After purification using an ExoSAP-IT PCR clean-up reagent (Affymetrix, Santa Clara, CA, USA), amplicons were sent to a commercial facility for sequencing (Macrogen, Amsterdam, the Netherlands). Sequences were aligned and edited using the DNASTAR Software 16 (Lasergene, Madison, WI, USA), and then compared to those available from the GenBank database using the BLAST algorithm. Obtained sequences were deposited in the GenBank database with accession numbers as follows: OK442622 for *A. proliferans*, OK442623 for *A. pseudoglaucus*, OK562707 for *A. chevalieri*, OK562740 for *A. cibarius*, OK442617 for *P. solitum*, OK442619 for *P. nalgiovense*, OK442616 for *P. citrinum*, OK442620 for *P. salamii*, OK442618 for *P. polonicum*, OK562705 for *P. oxalicum*, OK562706 for *P. bialowiezense* and OK442621 for *A. niger*.

2.4. Sensory Evaluation

Sensory evaluation of dry-cured ham samples was conducted by a trained panel of 9 assessors (5 males and 4 females) with an age range of 34 to 60 years (mean age = 49.3, SD = 8.9). The assessors were selected and generically trained according to [28]. In total, 13 training sessions of 60 min each took place. Basic training on how to use the scale and attribute generation based on the previous definitions [29] and attributes generated during training took place in the first four sessions. Nine training sessions were then held, during which panellists were trained on the quantification of the selected terms and calibration across assessors for improved consistency and reproducibility. Sensory analysis was carried out in the sensory laboratory of the Faculty of Food Technology and Biotechnology University of Zagreb according to [30] (room-related technical requirements: relative humidity 50–55%, temperature 20–22 °C) and illumination of 4000 K and 500 lux provided for the working table. Prior to sensory evaluation, assessors gave informed consent. Sensory evaluation made use of a quantitative descriptive analysis (QDA) based on the numerical and unipolar intensity scale developed in collaboration with the Centro Studi Assaggiatori (Brescia, Italy). The intensity of each sensory property was estimated using a numerical scale calibrated from left to right, with "0" indicating the absence of a given sensory property and "9" indicating its strongest intensity. Definitions and ranges of sensory traits are given in Table 1.

Individually coded samples were served at room temperature (two 1.5 mm-thick slices) in sensory booths. Samples were presented in a monadic manner in a randomised order and a 5 min break was taken between samples. In total, seven sessions were held over 4 days, and within each session five samples and one replicated sample were assessed. The replicated sample was used for the calculation of the assessor's repeatability (the calculation was based on the differences in absolute value between the scores assigned to the different descriptors of the sample and its replica) within Big Sensory Soft (Centro Studi Assaggiatori, Brescia, Italy). Water, yogurt, sour apple, and unsalted bread were provided to assessors between samples as palate cleansers. Sensory analysis embraced the assessment of visual qualities (colour of the muscle tissue, colour uniformity, colour of the subcutaneous adipose tissue—only for "Dalmatinski pršut", marbling, surface humidity, tyrosine crystals), olfactory qualities (favourable odour, unfavourable odour, smoky odour—only for "Dalmatinski pršut"), texture (tenderness, juiciness), mouth feel (saltiness, sweetness, sourness, bitterness) and aroma (specific aroma generated by aromatic herbs or butter, biochemical product properties, fresh meat aroma, moulds).

Table 1. Sensory traits, definitions and range implemented for sensory evaluation of dry-cured ham samples.

Sensory Traits	Definition (Range)
Appearance	
Colour of the muscle tissue	Intensity of red colour in the lean (pale pink to dark red)
Colour uniformity	Presence of colour homogeneity in the different muscles of a transversal cut (very low to very high)
Colour of the subcutaneous adipose tissue	Intensity of yellow colour of the fat (white to intense yellow)
Marbling	Level of visible intramuscular fat (very lean to intense marbled)
Surface humidity	Impresion of the surface wetness (very dry to very wet)
Tyrosine crystals	Presence of tyrosine crystals on the surface of a transversal cut (none to more than 10 crystals)
Odour	
Favourable odour	Intensity of the typical odour from cured meat products (very low to very high)
Unfavourable odour	Intensity of the off-odours (very low to very high)
Smoky odour	Perception of any type of smoke aroma (very low to very high)
Texture	
Tenderness	Effort required to bite thorough lean and to convert the sample to a swallowable state (very firm to very tender)
Juiciness	Impression of the release of juice during mastication (not to very juicy)
Taste	
Saltiness	Intensity of taste associated with sodium ions (not to very salty)
Sweetness	Intensity of sweetness (not to very sweet)
Sourness	Intensity of taste associated with citric acid (not to very sour)
Bitterness	Intensity of taste associated with caffeine (not to very bitter)
Aroma	
Specific aroma	Intensity of aroma associated with aromatic herbs (Istrian ham) and buttery aroma (Dalmatian ham) (very low to very high)
Biochemical aroma	Intensity of aroma associated with oxidised fat (very low to very high)
Fresh meat aroma	Intensity of aroma associated with fresh pork meat (very low to very high)
Moulds	Intensity of aroma associated with moulds (very low to very high)

2.5. Statistical Analysis

Statistical analyses were performed using the SPSS Statistics Software 22.0 (IBM, New York, NY, USA) and the Big Sensory Soft (Centro Studi Assaggiatori, Brescia, Italy). The results were tested for the normality of their distribution using the Shapiro–Wilk test. In order to determine the statistical significance of differences in sensory and mycological parameters between the two dry-cured hams coming from different regions, the independent samples t-test and Mann–Whitney U test were used. Decisions on statistical relevance were made at the significance level of $p < 0.05$. The results were subjected to principal component analysis (PCA) to interpret sensory attributes and mycological parameters of the two dry-cured hams using the Statistica 10.0 Software (StatSoft, Palo Alto, CA, USA).

3. Results and Discussion
3.1. The Presence of Mycobiota on Dry-Cured Ham Surface

The relative prevalence of mould strains growing on a dry-cured ham surface depends on the production area and technological production parameters. The latter include product ripening longevity, regional environmental conditions, temperature, and relative humidity during drying and ripening, and have a significant influence on home-based production during which these parameters are most often uncontrolled. The presence of moulds on the surface of dry-cured meat products is also dependent on physicochemical properties of the product, such as a_w, pH and salt content [9,31]. Given that the investigated types of dry-cured hams are protected at the national level in terms of protected geographical indication ("Dalmatinski pršut") and protected designation of origin ("Istarski pršut"), their production technologies are described in detail in Product Specifications [5,6]. The production of both types of dry-cured hams takes at least a year and is characterised by long-term ripening, yielding a finished product water activity (a_w) below 0.93 and a mass fraction of salt of 7.5% ("Dalmatinski pršut") and 8% ("Istarski pršut") at the maximum. These dry-cured hams are produced without inoculation of bacteria and mould starter cultures, so that wild moulds spontaneously overgrow their surfaces, despite continuous washing and brushing during the ripening period, intended to prevent an excessive mould growth. Earlier studies have shown that these products have characteristic pH values of less than 6.15 and less than 6.26, a_w below 0.89 and 0.85, and salt content of 6.0–9.2% and 6.0–9.8%, respectively [15,24,32]. Their ripening temperatures range from 12 to 19 °C [32], enabling the growth of species of the *Penicillium* and the *Aspergillus* genera [9,12].

Mould species identified on the surface of "Istarski pršut" and "Dalmatinski pršut" in this study are shown in Table 2.

Table 2. Surface mycobiota found on "Istarski pršut" and "Dalmatinski pršut".

Genus	Species	Number of Isolates	"Istarski Pršut" ($n = 15$)		"Dalmatinski Pršut" ($n = 20$)	
			Dr (%)	Fr (%)	Dr (%)	Fr (%)
Penicillium	P. salamii	6	9	43	-	-
	P. polonicum	2	3	14	-	-
	P. citrinum	14	9	43	12	40
	P. bialowienzense	4	6	29	-	-
	P. solitum	1	-	-	2	5
	P. nalgiovense	2	-	-	3	10
	P. oxalicum	2	-	-	3	10
Aspergillus	A. proliferans	14	13	64	8	25
	A. chevalieri	13	5	21	15	50
	A. pseudoglaucus	1	-	-	2	5
	A. niger	1	-	-	2	5
	A. cibarius	7	-	-	10	35

Dr (relative density) = the number of isolates of a given species/total number of isolates × 100. Fr = (relative frequency) the number of samples on which a given species was present/total number of samples × 100.

Examination of all dry-cured hams samples clearly shows that the species of the *Penicillium* and those of the *Aspergillus* genus are equally represented, given that 46% of the identified moulds were of the *Penicillium* and the remaining 54% of the *Aspergillus* genus, with no significant difference in the percentage of isolates between these two genera ($p = 0.346$). A total of 67 mould isolates and 12 different species (seven *Penicillium* and five *Aspergillus* species) were identified on 35 samples of both dry-cured ham types. The most represented species (listed together with the pertaining relative densities, Dr% = the number of isolates of a given species/total number of fungi isolated × 100) were *A.*

proliferans (Dr = 21%), *P. citrinum* (Dr = 21%) and *A. chevalieri* (Dr = 20%). These three species were the only ones found on the surfaces of both "Istarski pršut" and "Dalmatinski pršut". *P. citrinum* is generally taken to be one of most common fungal species on Earth, whereas citrinin conidiospores are one of the most common spores found in the air. Its ability to grow at a_w lower than 0.80 and a temperature of 5 °C helps this species to secure a niche in a wide range of habitats [33]. The highest prevalence of *A. chevalieri* and *A. proliferans* can be explained by the observation that the ascospores of *Aspergillus* teleomorphs can survive a wide range of temperatures (4–43 °C), and very low water activity (0.71) for up to 120 days. Moreover, *A. chevalieri* ranks as one of most common spoilage fungi on Earth, especially in warmer regions [26].

No statistically significant difference in the percentage of mould isolates between the two dry-cured ham types was found (p = 0.739) regardless of different production technology (smoked "Dalmatinski pršut"/non-smoked "Istarski pršut") and different climate in their production regions (hot Dalmatia vs. moderate climate Istria). Mycobiota on the surface of these products can be different depending on geographical and climate conditions; as the name itself says, "Istarski pršut" is produced in Istria and "Dalmatinski pršut" in Dalmatia. Dalmatia is a Croatian region known for its extremely hot and dry summers, often comparable to tropical and subtropical areas. In the hottest months, the day temperature frequently rises above 35 °C, whereas even in the coldest months it is maintained above 4 °C. Istria has a moderate Mediterranean climate, with a mean winter temperature in the coldest months of about 6 °C, and a mean summer temperature of 24 °C in the hottest months [5,6].

Similar results were obtained earlier by [12,34], who also failed to find any significant difference in the percentage of mould isolates found on the surfaces of smoked and non-smoked dry-fermented sausages and dry-cured hams coming from different Croatian regions. It was determined that 55% of mould isolates, among which 18% of the *Penicillium* and 37% of the *Aspergillus* genus, populate "Dalmatinski pršut", whereas 45% of isolates, among which 27% of the *Penicillium* and 18% of the *Aspergillus* genus, pertain to "Istarski pršut". A greater variety of *Aspergillus* species was observed with "Dalmatinski pršut" in comparison with "Istarski pršut", as also seen in a study by Zadravec et al. [12]. This was attributed to the climatic environment in which "Dalmatinski pršut" is produced, which is comparable to the subtropical and tropical areas that *Aspergillus* species prefer, contrary to *Penicillium* species, which favour lower environmental temperatures for their growth [26]. Earlier studies reported a decrease in the *Penicillium* population during ripening of dry-cured hams, whereas the *Aspergillus* population was isolated more frequently during post-drying and until the end-ripening phase, probably due to the higher resistance of its spores to drying of the air and ham, and increased temperature during summer ripening. Regarding the general number of mould isolates, at the end of the ripening period this was similar to that in the pre-ripening phase; the same result was found for the number of species [9,10].

"Dalmatinski pršut" showed a greater mould species diversity, with five *Aspergillus* and four *Penicillium* species identified, and the predominance of *A. chevalieri*, *P. citrinum* and *A. cibarius*. On the "Istarski pršut" surface, four *Penicillium* and only two *Aspergillus* species were identified, with the predominance of *A. proliferans*, *P. citrinum* and *P. salamii*. *A. cibarius*, *A. chevalieri* and *A. proliferans* belong to the resistant *Aspergillus* teleomorphs (*Eurotium*-type). *P. salamii* is closely related to the known starter culture *P. nalgiovense*, both species thereby occurring on cured meat products worldwide [35]. *P. salamii*, *P. polonicum* and *P. bialowienzense* were isolated only on "Istarski pršut", whereas *P. solitum*, *P. nalgiovense*, *P. oxalicum*, *A. pseudoglaucus*, *A. niger* and *A. cibarius* were found only on "Dalmatinski pršut". The diversity of species colonising "Istarski pršut" and "Dalmatinski pršut" can also be attributed to the different environment around ripening chambers from which mould spores mostly come, in addition to the ripening conditions in these chambers, because homemade dry-cured hams often ripen uncontrolled [8]. This should also be taken into account when comparing the species identified in this study to the mould species found to be predominant in other studies of "Dalmatinski pršut" and "Istarski pršut" [9,12] or dry-cured hams from other countries [8,10,31,36].

To the best to our knowledge, only two studies have been conducted on surface mycobiota of these two types of dry-cured hams, as a part of the PDO or the PGI denominations [9,12]. In the research of "Dalmatinski pršut" and "Istarski pršut" by Zadravec et al. [12], a higher number of species (19–20) was identified in comparison with this study (9–12). In both ham types, the dominating species were *P. solitum, P. nalgiovense, P. commune,* and *P. polonicum*. With the exception of *P. commune*, the species mentioned above were also found on ham surfaces in this study, but not as dominating ones. In that research [12], *P. citrinum* was found only occasionally in comparison with this study. Regarding the species of the *Aspergillus* genus, in addition to *A. proliferans, A. pseudoglaucus,* and toxigenic *A. niger*, in the research by Zadravec et al. [12] *A. versicolor* and *A. ochraceus* were also isolated; however, *Aspergillus* sp. were isolated less frequently and not as predominant species, as opposed to the present research. In the study of Istrian ham by Comi et al. [9], the most frequently isolated species were *P. frequentas, P. verrucosum, P. lanosocoeruleum, P. chrysogenum, P. commune* and *P. expansum,* but these species were identified using traditional rather than molecular methods.

In contrast to our research, the dominant mould species found on hams originating from other European countries—for example, *P. commune* and *P. chrysogenum* found on Spanish hams such as the Iberian prosciutto [36,37]—were not identified in the present study. The Italian ham San Daniele was reported to harbour *P. chrysogenum* and *A. fumigatus* [10], whereas the Norwegian hams were found to host *P. nalgiovense, P. solitum* and *P. commune* [31]. Slovenian hams were claimed to harbour *P. nordicum, P. nalgiovense* and *P. milanense* [11]. In general, the higher representation and greater diversity of *Aspergillus* species found in our research can be explained by the fact that Istrian, and especially Dalmatian, prosciuttos ripen in warmer and drier climates compared to the prosciuttos investigated in the studies quoted above. Moulds can influence the sensory properties of dry-cured hams, such as their surface coverage and appearance. Moulds can imbue a favourable white or greyish fungal coverage, which is deemed to be produced by *P. salamii* and *P. nalgiovense*, whereas brown/green sporulation and black spot formation are deemed to be signs of spoilage. The study of sausages inoculated with *P. salamii* and *P. nalgiovense* evidenced a higher favourable contribution of *P. salamii* to sausage coverage, appearance, and flavour, compared to that of *P. nalgiovense* [14,37]. Due to their enzymatic activity, moulds contribute to the nascence of volatile compounds; however, the results of the study by Martín et al. [14] showed that the differences in volatile compounds produced by different fungal populations do not impact the flavour score of the sensory analysis but enhance the overall acceptability due to the improved texture.

It is known that some of the surface moulds can produce mycotoxins as their secondary metabolites, which can have a number of adverse effects on human and animal health [20,35]. In previous research of Croatian dry-fermented meat products, contamination with ochratoxin A (OTA), citrinin (CIT), aflatoxin B1 (AFB_1) and cyclopiazonic acid (CPA) was evidenced [20,38–40], consistent with other types of dry-cured meat products originating from other countries [41–44]. The mycotoxigenic mould species identified in this study were *Penicillium citrinum* as a CIT-producer, *Penicillium polonicum* as a verrucosidin and nephrotoxic glycopeptides producer, and *Aspergillus niger* as an OTA producer. "Dalmatinski pršut" and "Istarski pršut" surfaces hosted a similar percentage of mycotoxigenic species (14% and 12%, respectively).

3.2. The Effect of Surface Mycobiota on Sensory Properties

The results of the sensory evaluation of "Istarski pršut" and "Dalmatinski pršut" and quantitative descriptive analysis are shown in Figure 1.

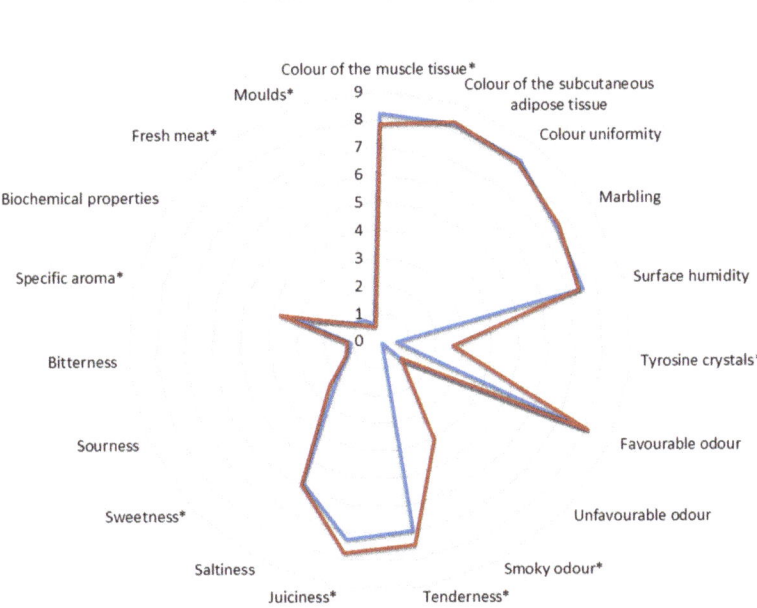

Figure 1. Sensory characteristics of "Istarski pršut" and "Dalmatinski pršut" (appearance, odour, texture, taste, and aroma). * statistically significant difference; numerical scale of intensity of sensory properties: "0" indicates the absence of a given sensory property, and "9" indicates its strongest intensity.

Statistical analysis revealed significant differences ($p < 0.05$) between "Istarski pršut" and "Dalmatinski pršut" in 9 of 20 attributes. The differences were found in visual qualities, odour, texture, taste, and aroma, as follows: colour of the muscle tissue ($p < 0.001$), tyrosine crystals ($p < 0.001$), smoky odour ($p < 0.001$), tenderness ($p < 0.001$), juiciness ($p < 0.001$), sweetness ($p = 0.004$), specific aromas ($p = 0.048$), fresh meat aroma ($p = 0.001$) and mould aroma ($p = 0.047$).

In terms of appearance, significant variations were found in the colour of the muscle tissue and tyrosine crystals content, where "Istarski pršut" had a more intense muscle colour and lower tyrosine crystals content. According to the Product Specifications, visual characteristics of "Istarski pršut" and "Dalmatinski pršut" should embrace evenly red to bright red muscle tissue colour; white to pink-white subcutaneous adipose tissue in "Dalmatinski pršut; and a lack of skin and subcutaneous adipose tissue in "Istarski pršut" [5,6]. "Istarski pršut" is allowed to be produced from raw hams obtained from pigs older than 9 months, having a live weight of at least 160 kg. The fulfilment of these requirements results in a higher myoglobin meat content [45] that affects the muscle colour. Furthermore, in dry-cured hams, salt diffusions play an important role in the development of colour, whereas surface moulds can stabilise it. However, diverse factors of other natures can also affect meat colour, such as fermentation time, smoking, and storage [46]. Tyrosine crystals are formed in a ham due to long ripening, which enhances the precipitation of the amino acid tyrosine responsible for white spot appearance, also indicating possible longer maturation and more intense proteolysis [47] that can be enhanced by surface moulds.

Acceptability of dry-cured hams is also highly dependent on texture parameters. According to the Product Specifications, "Dalmatinski pršut" should have a soft chewy consistency, whereas hard consistency and minimal solubility are deemed unacceptable [6]. Tenderness and juiciness of "Dalmatinski pršut" scored significantly higher than those of

"Istarski pršut". The study of Martín et al. [14] showed that the softer texture of inoculated dry-cured hams is a direct consequence of mould inoculation. An early settling of moulds on hams prevents excessive drying of the surface, thus lowering dryness. In addition, proteolysis increased by moulds contributes to lower toughness. Ludemann et al. [48] showed inter- and intra- mould species differences in proteolytic activities, and that the addition of salt stimulates proteolytic activity of mould strains at 25 °C. *P. nalgiovense*, which was found on "Dalmatinski pršut", is known for its proteolytic activity [8,17]. Proteolysis increased by surface moulds may explain the greater tenderness of "Dalmatinski pršut".

The "Istarski pršut" Product Specifications require that the product should have a mild, moderately salty taste, whereas "Dalmatinski pršut" is expected to have a mildly saltish or salty taste; an overly salty or sour/bitter taste, or an entangled and undefinable mixture of tastes, are not allowed [5,6]. Significant variations between the products under study were only found for their sweetness, "Dalmatinski pršut" being sweeter than "Istarski pršut". The overall saltiness of the products was characterised as moderate (5.8–5.9), whereas sweetness, sourness and bitterness achieved low scores (2.1–2.5, 1.2–1.3, and 1.1–1.2, respectively). In the research by Petričević et al. [4], the sweetness of "Istarski pršut" was more pronounced than that of "Dalmatinski pršut". Volatile compounds, such as 2-ethyl furane, 2-pentanone, heptane and octane contribute to the sensory perceptions of sweetness [49]. In the study of "Istarski pršut" by Marušić et al. [23], sweetness and the presence of esters formed by esterification of carboxylic acids and alcohols were positively correlated (the higher the concentrations of esters, the more pronounced the sweetness of the product). Studies have confirmed the ability of *Mucor* and *Penicillium* strains to produce esters [19]. In the study by Bruna et al. [50], the highest levels of esters were detected in superficially inoculated sausages in comparison with uninoculated control sausages, which indicates the contribution of mould metabolic activity to the sweetness of a product.

A salty taste is the result of addition of sodium chloride in the salting stage, whereas a bitter taste is the result of vivid proteolysis, which generates free hydrophobic amino acids and peptides responsible for the taste. A sour taste also originates from amino acids and short free fatty acids produced during proteolysis and lipolysis [51]. Martín et al. [16] showed higher concentrations of some polar amino acids (Asp, Glu, HIs, Thr, Arg and Pro) in inoculated dry-cured hams, as opposed to Iberian hams overgrown by an uncontrolled fungal population. Conversely, some less polar amino acids (Ile, Leu and Trp) were shown to be less present in inoculated hams than in those overgrown by an uncontrolled fungal population. A higher polar/lipophilic free amino acids' ratio is considered flavour-enhancing due to the high correlation between bitterness and lipophilic free amino acids [16]. For the sake of clarity, the comparison with the results of studies devoted to inoculated dry-cured meat products implies meat inoculation with species having beneficial effects, such as *P. chrysogenum*, *P. nalgiovense*, *P. aurantiogriseum*, *P. camemberti*, *P. salamii* and *P. solitum* [13,16,48,50,52].

A smoky odour was reported only for "Dalmatinski pršut", which achieved a score of 4.06. A smoky aroma represents the most distinctive feature of "Dalmatinski pršut" compared to other types of dry-cured hams produced in the broader region; the feature in question makes the product easiest to recognise, whereas the Product Specifications require this odour to be just mild [6]. Phenolic compounds are mainly responsible for the unique aroma and taste of smoked products; in the research of volatile compounds of Croatian dry-cured hams, 18 phenols were identified in smoked dry-cured hams, whereas unsmoked products contained 4-methylphenol only [4].

A specific aroma can be developed from aromatic herbs or butter. It has been shown that terpenes are positively correlated with the flavour coming from added herbal spices, such as pepper and rosemary, which are added in the salting phase of "Istarski pršut" production [23]. For the specific buttery aroma, ketones, such as 2,3 butanedione, are responsible [51]. The "Dalmatinski pršut" Product Specifications require the product to have pleasant aromas of fermented, salted, dry and smoked pig meat, and to be free of any strange odours (such as tar, oil, fresh meat, wet or dry grass odours) [6]. Mouldy and fresh meat aromas were significantly more pronounced in the case of "Istarski pršut", but these attributes, together with biochemical properties, generally scored very low (0.5–0.6; 0.7–0.9 and <1.1, respectively). A fresh meat aroma is more pronounced with shorter-ripened products, so that the differences in fresh meat aroma score between "Istarski pršut" and "Dalmatinski pršut" can be attributed to the shorter ripening of "Dalmatinski pršut" [23]. In addition, active fungal metabolism of lipophilic amino acids increases the content of volatile compounds related to these amino acids, such as branched aldehydes and carboxylic acids associated with the distinct flavour of dry-cured, long-maturing and aged products. Therefore, the differences in fresh pork meat aroma between "Istarski pršut" and "Dalmatinski pršut" may also be the result of a more vivid metabolic mould activity taking place on the surface of "Dalmatinski pršut", thus generating lipophilic amino acids, and, consequently, the volatile compounds mentioned above [16].

To determine the relationship between sensory traits and surface moulds of the two types of dry-cured ham, PCA analysis was performed, as shown in Figures 2 and 3.

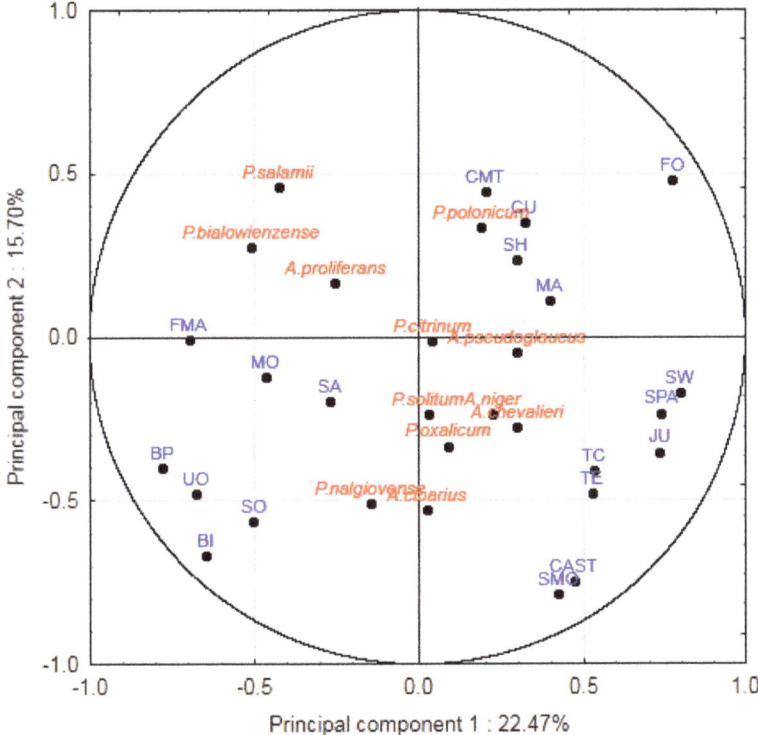

Figure 2. Score plot of the variables encompassed by the principal component analysis of sensory attributes and mould species of "Istarski pršut" and "Dalmatinski pršut". CMT = colour of the muscle tissue; CAST = colour of the subcutaneous adipose tissue; CU = colour uniformity; MA = marbling; SH = surface humidity; TC = tyrosine crystals; FO = favourable odour; UO = unfavourable odour; SMO = smoky odour; TE = tenderness; JU = juiciness; SA = saltiness; SW = sweetness; SO = sourness; BI = bitterness; SPA = specific aroma; BP = biochemical properties; FMA = fresh meat aroma; MO = moulds.

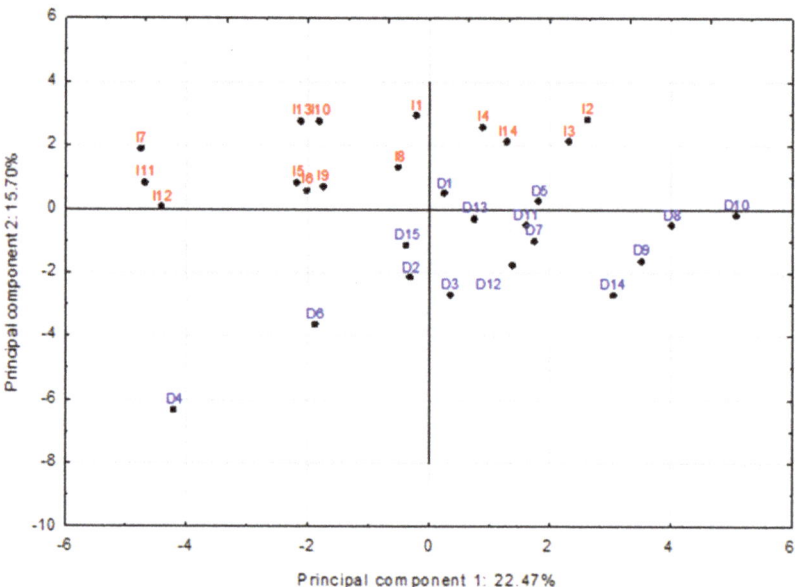

Figure 3. Score plot of the principal component analysis of the sensory attributes and mould species of "Istarski pršut" (I) and "Dalmatinski pršut" (D) samples.

The measurements and PCs were interpreted based on the correlations between each parameter and each PC. Thus, variables that were close to each other were considered positively correlated, those separated by 180° as negatively correlated, and those separated by 90° as independently correlated. As can be seen in Figure 2, which shows the relationship between variables, favourable odour, sweetness, specific aroma, and juiciness were the main contributors to the positive side, whereas biochemical aroma and fresh meat aroma, unfavourable odour, and bitterness accounted for the negative side of PC1. This is also an indication of a strong negative correlation between the desired and undesired sensory properties, as established for artisanal smoked dry-cured ham by Kos et al. [53]. Similar results were achieved by Pham et al. [29], who presented sweetness on one side, and bitterness and biochemical aroma on the other, of the same principal component. The same authors reported that saltiness and cured flavour were close to each other and to the bitterness and rancid aroma, indicating a positive correlation between them, but this was not observed in the present research.

The positive side of PC2 was mostly correlated to the colour of the muscle tissue and colour uniformity. In addition to the smoky odour and the colour of the subcutaneous adipose tissue (characteristic only for "Dalmatinski pršut"), the most important variables on the negative side of PC2 were bitterness and sourness, suggesting a strong positive correlation between the two. Although mould aroma, tyrosine crystals and tenderness of the two ham types were significantly different, their correlation with the principal component arrangement was weak, as was the contribution of marbling, saltiness, and surface humidity. Interestingly, mould species were correlated to PC2, for which the closest relationship of *P. polonicum* and *P. salamii* was established on the positive side, whereas the major contributors to the negative side were *P. cibarius* and *P. nalgiovense*. It was found that other mould species were not important for the characterisation of the first two principal components. However, it was found that *P. polonicum* was closely related to the colour of the muscle tissue, colour uniformity and surface humidity, suggesting a high correlation between them and a possible favourable effect of that mould species on the development of the sensory traits in question.

In the score plot on Figure 3, a clear separation between "Istarski pršut" and "Dalmatinski pršut" samples along PC2 can be observed. "Istarski pršut" samples occupy the upper quadrants of the positive and the negative side of PC1, where the colour of the muscle tissue and colour uniformity, in addition to two mould species (*P. salamii* and *P. polonicum*), made the highest contribution. "Istarski pršut" samples occupy the upper quadrants of the positive and the negative side of the PC1, where the colour of the muscle tissue and colour uniformity, in addition to two mould species (*P. salamii* and *P. polonicum*), made the highest contribution. By comparison, "Dalmatinski pršut" samples dominantly occupy the lower quadrants of the positive and the negative side of PC1, where the sensory traits smoky odour, colour of the subcutaneous adipose tissue and bitterness, and the mould species *P. nalgiovense* and *A. cibarius*, were considered important. Furthermore, it was found that *P. salamii*, *P. bialowienzense*, *P. polonicum* and *A. proliferans* were closely related to the "Istarski pršut" samples, whereas *P. nalgiovense*, *A. cibarius*, *P. oxalicum*, *A. niger*, *A. chevalieri* and *P. solitum* were related to the "Dalmatinski pršut" samples. Therefore, it can be concluded that mould species are an important source of information needed for better ham characterisation.

4. Conclusions

The study results showed no significant differences in the number of mould isolates between "Istarski pršut" and "Dalmatinski pršut", produced using different production technologies (smoked/non-smoked) and coming from different climatic regions, but did show species diversity, and higher percentage and greater variety of *Aspergillus* species in "Dalmatinski pršut". Different conditions under which dry-cured hams are processed, and consequently different moulds that develop on their surface, resulted in significant variations in 9 of 20 sensory attributes. Predominant species found on the surface of "Dalmatinski pršut" were *A. chevalieri*, *P. citrinum* and *A. cibarius*, whereas those predominating on the surface of "Istarski pršut" were *A. proliferans*, *P. citrinum* and *P. salamii*. A more pronounced tenderness and juiciness, higher tyrosine crystals content, and lesser fresh meat aroma can indicate higher proteolytic activities of mould species populating the surface of "Dalmatinski pršut" in comparison with "Istarski pršut". The results of the PCA analysis indicated that several sensory traits appeared to be important for ham type distinction. Based on the PCA analysis, mould species are primarily correlated with the second principal component, for which the ham types were clearly separated. Furthermore, different mould species were loaded close to each dry-cured ham type, and are thus a significant source of information needed for better ham characterisation.

Author Contributions: Conceptualization, T.L. and J.P.; methodology, I.K., N.V. and M.Z.; software, I.K., N.V. and T.L.; validation, I.K. and N.V.; formal analysis, I.K., N.V., I.P., M.Z. and T.L.; investigation, I.K., N.V., I.P., T.L. and M.Z.; resources, D.M. and E.L.; data curation, N.V., I.K. and T.L.; writing—original draft preparation, T.L.; writing—review and editing, J.P.; visualization, T.L. and J.P.; supervision, J.P.; project administration, J.P.; funding acquisition, J.P. All authors have read and agreed to the published version of the manuscript.

Funding: This research was funded by the Croatian Science Foundation under the project "Mycotoxins in traditional Croatian meat products: molecular identification of mycotoxin-producing moulds and consumer exposure assessment" (No. IP-2018-01-9017).

Data Availability Statement: The sequences of mould isolates included in this study are openly, available in GenBank with accession numbers as described in the Section 2.

Conflicts of Interest: The authors declare no conflict of interest.

References

1. Benedini, R.; Parolari, G.; Toscani, T.; Virgili, R. Sensory and texture properties of Italian typical dry-cured hams as related to maturation time and salt content. *Meat Sci.* **2012**, *90*, 431–437. [CrossRef] [PubMed]
2. Flores, M. Sensory descriptors for dry-cured meat products. In *Sensory Analysis of Foods of Animal Origin*; Nolet, L.M., Toldra, F., Eds.; CRC Press: Boca Raton, FL, USA, 2011; pp. 173–192.

3. García-González, D.L.; Roncales, P.; Cilla, I.; Del Río, S.; Poma, J.P.; Aparicio, R. Interlaboratory evaluation of dry-cured hams (from France and Spain) by assessors from two different nationalities. *Meat Sci.* **2006**, *73*, 521–528. [CrossRef] [PubMed]
4. Petričević, S.; Marušić Radovčić, N.; Lukić, K.; Listeš, E.; Medić, H. Differentiation of dry-cured hams from different processing methods by means of volatile compounds, physico-chemical and sensory analysis. *Meat Sci.* **2018**, *137*, 217–227. [CrossRef] [PubMed]
5. Ministry of Agriculture. Product Specification "Istarski Pršut"/"Istrski Pršut" for Registration of Protected Designation of Origin. 2014. Available online: https://poljoprivreda.gov.hr/UserDocsImages/arhiva/datastore/filestore/97/Izmijenjena_Specifikacija_proizvoda_Istarski_prsut-Istrski_prsut.pdf (accessed on 4 January 2021).
6. Ministry of Agriculture. Product Specification "Dalmatinski Pršut" for Registration of Protected Geographical Indications. 2015. Available online: https://www.prsut-vostane.hr/hr/specifikacija-dalmatinski-prsut.pdf (accessed on 11 January 2021).
7. Prado, N.; Sampayo, M.; González, P.; Lombó, F.; Díaz, J. Physicochemical, sensory and microbiological characterization of Asturian Chorizo, a traditional fermented sausage manufactured in Northern Spain. *Meat Sci.* **2019**, *156*, 118–124. [CrossRef]
8. Alapont, C.; Martinez-Culebras, P.V.; Lopez-Mendoza, M.C. Determination of lipolytic and proteolytic activities of mycoflora isolated from dry-cured teruel ham. *J. Food Sci. Technol.* **2014**, *52*, 5250–5256. [CrossRef]
9. Comi, G.; Orlić, S.; Redžepović, S.; Urso, R.; Iacumin, L. Moulds isolated from Istrian dried ham at the pre-ripening and ripening level. *Int. J. Food Microbiol.* **2004**, *96*, 29–34. [CrossRef]
10. Comi, G.; Iacumin, L. Ecology of moulds during the pre-ripening and ripening of San Daniele dry cured ham. *Food Res. Int.* **2013**, *54*, 1113–1119. [CrossRef]
11. Sonjak, S.; Ličen, M.; Frisvald, J.C.; Gunde-Cimerman, N. The mycobiota of three dry-cured meat products from Slovenia. *Food Microbiol.* **2011**, *28*, 373–376. [CrossRef]
12. Zadravec, M.; Vahčić, N.; Brnić, D.; Markov, K.; Frece, J.; Beck, R.; Lešić, T.; Pleadin, J. A study of surface moulds and mycotoxins in Croatian traditional dry-cured meat products. *Int. J. Food Microbiol.* **2020**, *317*, 108459. [CrossRef]
13. Magista, D.; Susca, A.; Ferrara, M.; Logrieco, A.F.; Perrone, G. *Penicillium* species: Crossroad between quality and safety of cured meat production. *Curr. Opin. Food Sci.* **2017**, *17*, 36–40. [CrossRef]
14. Martín, A.; Córdoba, J.J.; Aranda, E.; Córdoba, M.G.; Asensio, M.A. Contribution of a selected fungal population to the volatile compounds on dry-cured ham. *Int. J. Food Microbiol.* **2006**, *110*, 8–18. [CrossRef]
15. Marušić, N.; Petrović, M.; Vidaček, S.; Petrak, T.; Medić, H. Characterization of traditional Istrian dry-cured ham by means of physical and chemical analyses and volatile compounds. *Meat Sci.* **2011**, *88*, 786–790. [CrossRef]
16. Martín, A.; Córdoba, J.J.; Núñez, F.; Benito, M.J.; Asensio, M.A. Contribution of a selected fungal population to proteolysis on dry-cured ham. *Int. J. Food Microbiol.* **2004**, *94*, 55–66. [CrossRef]
17. Garcia, M.; Casas, C.; Toledo, V.; Selgas, M.D. Effect of selected mould strains on the sensory properties of dry fermented sausages. *Eur. Food Res. Technol.* **2001**, *212*, 287–291. [CrossRef]
18. Ockerman, H.W.; Céspedes Sánchez, F.J.; León Crespo, F. Influence of molds on flavor quality of Spanish ham. *J. Muscle Foods* **2000**, *11*, 247–259. [CrossRef]
19. Sunesen, L.O.; Stahnke, L.H. Mould starter cultures for dry sausages-selection, application and effects. *Meat Sci.* **2003**, *65*, 935–948. [CrossRef]
20. Pleadin, J.; Zadravec, M.; Brnić, D.; Perković, I.; Škrivanko, M.; Kovačević, D. Moulds and mycotoxins detected in the regional speciality fermented sausage 'slavonski kulen' during a 1-year production period. *Food Addit. Contam. A* **2017**, *34*, 282–290. [CrossRef]
21. Sunesen, L.O.; Trihaas, J.; Stahnke, L.H. Volatiles in a sausage surface model-influence of *Penicillium nalgiovense, Pediococcus pentosaceus*, ascorbate, nitrate and temperature. *Meat Sci.* **2004**, *66*, 447–456. [CrossRef]
22. Jerković, I.; Mastelić, J.; Tartaglia, S. A study of volatile flavour substances in Dalmatian traditional smoked ham: Impact of dry-curing and frying. *Food Chem.* **2007**, *104*, 1030–1039. [CrossRef]
23. Marušić, N.; Vidaček, S.; Janči, T.; Petrak, T.; Medić, H. Determination of volatile compounds and quality parameters of traditional Istrian dry-cured ham. *Meat Sci.* **2014**, *96*, 1409–1416. [CrossRef]
24. Marušić Radovčić, N.; Vidaček, S.; Janči, T.; Medić, H. Characterization of volatile compounds, physico-chemical and sensory characteristics of smoked dry-cured ham. *J. Food Sci. Technol.* **2016**, *53*, 4093–4105. [CrossRef]
25. Pleadin, J.; Lešić, T.; Vahčić, N.; Raspović, I.; Malenica Staver, M.; Krešić, G.; Bogdanović, T.; Kovačević, D. Seasonal variations in fatty acids composition of Istrian and Dalmatian prosciutto. *Meso* **2015**, *5*, 449–454.
26. Pitt, J.I.; Hocking, A.D. *Fungi and Food Spoilage*; Springer: New York, NY, USA, 2009.
27. Samson, R.A.; Houbraken, J.; Thrane, U.; Frisvad, J.C.; Andersen, B. *Food and Indoor Fungi*, 2nd ed.; Westerdijk Fungal Biodiversity Institute: Utrecht, The Netherlands, 2019.
28. International Organization for Standardization (ISO). *Sensory Analysis-Methodology-Guidelines for Monitoring the Performance of a Quantitative Sensory Panel*; ISO Standard 11132:2012; ISO: Geneva, Switzerland, 2012.
29. Pham, A.J.; Schilling, M.W.; Mikel, W.B.; Williams, J.B.; Martin, J.M.; Coggins, P.C. Relationships between sensory descriptors, consumer acceptability and volatile flavor compounds of American dry-cured ham. *Meat Sci.* **2008**, *80*, 728–737. [CrossRef]
30. ISO. *Guidance for the Design of Test Rooms*; ISO Standard 8589:2007; ISO: Geneva, Switzerland, 2007.
31. Asefa, D.T.; Gjerde, R.O.; Sidhu, M.S.; Langsrud, S.; Kure, C.F.; Nesbakken, T.; Skaar, I. Moulds contaminants on Norwegian dry-cured meat products. *Int. J. Food Microbiol.* **2009**, *128*, 435–439. [CrossRef]

32. Kovačević, D. *Kemija i Tehnologija Šunki i Pršuta*; Prehrambeno-Tehnološki Fakultet: Osijek, Croatia, 2017.
33. Geisen, R.; Schmidt-Heydt, M.; Touhami, N.; Himmelsbach, A. New aspects of ochratoxin A and citrinin biosynthesis in *Penicillium*. *Curr. Opin. Food Sci.* **2018**, *23*, 23–31. [CrossRef]
34. Lešić, T.; Vahčić, N.; Kos, I.; Zadravec, M.; Sinčić Pulić, B.; Bogdanović, T.; Petričević, S.; Listeš, E.; Škrivanko, M.; Pleadin, J. Characterization of Traditional Croatian Household-Produced Dry-Fermented Sausages. *Foods* **2020**, *9*, 990. [CrossRef]
35. Perrone, G.; Samson, R.A.; Frisvad, J.C.; Susca, A.; Gunde-Cimerman, N.; Epifani, F.; Houbraken, J. *Penicillium salamii*, a new species occurring during seasoning of dry-cured meat. *Int. J. Food Microbiol.* **2015**, *193*, 91–98. [CrossRef]
36. Alapont, C.; López-Mendoza, M.C.; Gil, J.V.; Martínez-Culebras, P.V. Mycobiota and toxigenic *Penicillium* species on two Spanish dry-cured ham manufacturing plants. *Food Addit. Contam. A* **2014**, *31*, 93–104. [CrossRef]
37. Núñez, F.; Rodríguez, M.M.; Bermúdez, M.E.; Córdoba, J.J.; Asensio, M.A. Composition and toxigenic potential of the mould population on dry-cured Iberian ham. *Int. J. Food Microbiol.* **1996**, *32*, 185–197. [CrossRef]
38. Markov, K.; Pleadin, J.; Bevardi, M.; Vahčić, N.; Sokolić-Mihalek, D.; Frece, J. Natural occurrence of aflatoxin B_1, ochratoxin A and citrinin in Croatian fermented meat products. *Food Control* **2013**, *34*, 312–317. [CrossRef]
39. Vulić, A.; Lešić, T.; Kudumija, N.; Zadravec, M.; Kiš, M.; Vahčić, N.; Pleadin, J. The development of LC-MS/MS method of determination of cyclopiazonic acid in dry-fermented meat products. *Food Control* **2020**, *123*, 107814. [CrossRef]
40. Pleadin, J.; Malenica Staver, M.; Vahčić, N.; Kovačević, D.; Milone, S.; Saftić, L.; Scortichini, G. Survey of aflatoxin B^1 and ochratoxin A occurrence in traditional meat products coming from Croatian households and markets. *Food Control* **2015**, *52*, 71–77. [CrossRef]
41. Iacumin, L.; Milesi, S.; Pirani, S.; Comi, G.; Chiesa, L.M. Ochratoxigenic mold and ochratoxin a in fermented sausages from different areas in Northern Italy: Occurrence, reduction or prevention with ozonated air. *J. Food Saf.* **2011**, *31*, 538–545. [CrossRef]
42. Montanha, F.M.; Anater, A.; Burchard, J.F.; Luciano, F.L.; Meca, G.; Manyes, L.; Pimpão, C.T. Mycotoxins in dry-cured meats: A review. *Food Chem. Toxicol.* **2018**, *111*, 494–502. [CrossRef] [PubMed]
43. Peromingo, B.; Rodríguez, M.; Núñez, F.; Silva, A.; Rodríguez, A. Sensitive determination of cyclopiazonic acid in dry-cured ham using a QuEChERS method and UHPLC–MS/MS. *Food Chem.* **2018**, *263*, 275–282. [CrossRef] [PubMed]
44. Rodrigues, P.; Silva, D.; Costa, P.; Abrunhosa, L.; Venancio, A.; Teixeira, A. Mycobiota and mycotoxins in Portuguese pork, goat and sheep dry-cured hams. *Mycotoxin Res.* **2019**, *35*, 405–412. [CrossRef] [PubMed]
45. Ortiz, A.; García-Torres, S.; González, E.; De Pedro-Sanz, E.J.; Gaspar, P.; Tejerina, D. Quality traits of fresh and dry-cured loin from Iberian × Duroc crossbred pig in the Montanera system according to slaughtering age. *Meat Sci.* **2020**, *170*, 108242. [CrossRef]
46. Perez-Alvarez, J.A.; Fernandez-Lopez, J. Color Characteristic of Meat and poultry processing. In *Sensory Analysis of Foods of Animal Origin*; Nolet, L.M., Toldra, F., Eds.; CRC Press: Boca Raton, FL, USA, 2011; pp. 101–113.
47. Toldra, F. *Dry-Cured Meat Products*; Food and Nutrition Press: Trumbull, CT, USA, 2002.
48. Ludemann, V.; Pose, G.; Pollio, M.L.; Segura, J. Determination of growth characteristics and lipolytic and proteolytic activities of *Penicillium* strains isolated from Argentinean salami. *Int. J. Food Microbiol.* **2004**, *96*, 13–18. [CrossRef]
49. García-González, D.L.; Tena, N.; Aparicio-Ruiz, R.; Morales, M.T. Relationship between sensory attributes and volatile compounds qualifying dry-cured hams. *Meat Sci.* **2008**, *80*, 315–325. [CrossRef]
50. Bruna, J.M.; Hierro, E.M.; De la Hoz, L.; Mottram, D.S.; Fernández, M.; Ordóñez, J.A. The contribution of *Penicillium aurantiogriseum* to the volatile composition and sensory quality of dry fermented sausages. *Meat Sci.* **2001**, *59*, 97–107. [CrossRef]
51. Flores, M. Flavour of meat products. In *Sensory Analysis of Foods of Animal Origin*; Nolet, L.M., Toldra, F., Eds.; CRC Press: Boca Raton, FL, USA, 2011; pp. 131–143.
52. Bruna, J.M.; Hierro, E.M.; De la Hoz, L.; Mottram, D.S.; Fernández, M.; Ordóñez, J.A. Changes in selected biochemical and sensory parameters as affected by the superficial inoculation of *Penicillium camemberti* on dry fermented sausages. *Int. J. Food Microbiol.* **2003**, *85*, 111–125. [CrossRef]
53. Kos, I.; Sinčić Pulić, B.; Gorup, D.; Kaić, A. Sensory profiles of artisanal smoked dry-cured ham as affected by production season. *J. Cent. Eur. Agric.* **2019**, *20*, 1089–1098. [CrossRef]

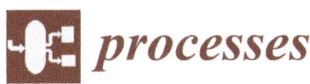

Article

Antimicrobial Resistance of *Lactobacillus johnsonii* and *Lactobacillus zeae* in Raw Milk

Jana Výrostková, Ivana Regecová *, Mariana Kováčová, Slavomír Marcinčák, Eva Dudriková and Jana Maľová

Department of Food Hygiene, Technology and Safety, The University of Veterinary Medicine and Pharmacy in Košice, Komenského 73, 041 81 Košice, Slovakia; jana.vyrostkova@uvlf.sk (J.V.); mariana.kovacova@student.uvlf.sk (M.K.); slavomir.marcincak@uvlf.sk (S.M.); eva.dudrikova@uvlf.sk (E.D.); jana.malova@uvlf.sk (J.M.)
* Correspondence: ivana.regecova@uvlf.sk

Received: 18 November 2020; Accepted: 8 December 2020; Published: 10 December 2020

Abstract: *Lactobacillus johnsonii* and *Lactobacillus zeae* are among the lactobacilli with probiotic properties, which occur in sour milk products, cheeses, and to a lesser extent in raw milk. Recently, resistant strains have been detected in various species of lactobacilli. The aim of the study was to determine the incidence of resistant *Lactobacillus johnsonii* and *Lactobacillus zeae* strains in various types of raw milk. A total of 245 isolates were identified by matrix-assisted laser desorption/ionization mass spectrometry and polymerase chain reaction methods as *Lactobacillus* sp., of which 23 isolates of *Lactobacillus johnsonii* and 18 isolates of *Lactobacillus zeae* were confirmed. Determination of susceptibility to selected antibiotics was performed using the E-test and broth dilution method, where 7.3% of lactobacilli strains were evaluated as ampicillin-resistant, 14.7% of isolates as erythromycin-resistant, and 4.9% of isolates as clindamycin-resistant. The genus *Lactobacillus johnsonii* had the highest resistance to erythromycin (34.8%), similar to *Lactobacillus zeae* (33.3%). Of the 41 isolates, the presence of the gene was confirmed in five *Lactobacillus johnsonii* strains and in two strains of *Lactobacillus zeae*. The presence of resistant strains of *Lactobacillus johnsonii* and *Lactobacillus zeae* is a potential risk in terms of spreading antimicrobial resistance through the food chain.

Keywords: antimicrobial resistance; *Lactobacillus johnsonii*; *Lactobacillus zeae*; MALDI-TOF-MS; milk; PCR

1. Introduction

Lactobacilli belonging to the family Lactobacillaceae are one of the most important bacteria found in the dairy industry. Due to their beneficial effects, they are often used for the production of fermented foods or as probiotics [1,2]. Among them we include the so-called wild lactobacilli, such as *Lactobacillus (Lb.) paracasei*, *Lb. praplantarum*, *Lb. plantarum*, and *Lb. johnsonii*, which have antimicrobial as well as probiotic properties. The most common lactobacillus in fermented milk is *Lb. johnsonii* [3,4]. *Lb. johnsonii* is characterized by processing and protective properties in the production of cheese and beverages. *Lb. johnsonii* also have good potential probiotic properties, especially in terms of lysozyme resistance and simulated gastric juice environment [5]. Another important species of lactobacilli is *Lactobacillus zeae*, which is responsible for the hydrolysis of a cow's milk protein [6]. It has a strong inhibitory effect on angiotensin converting enzyme (ACE) [7]. These species are found to a lesser extent in raw milk. Their number increases mainly during the production of dairy products. We rank these lactobacilli among non-starting lactic acid bacteria (LAB) [8].

Recently, lactobacilli, as well as other LAB, have been detected as a potential reservoir of antimicrobial resistance in the food chain [9], which has also been confirmed by the presence of resistant LAB strains (including lactobacilli) in the most-consumed fermented foods [10,11]. Lactobacilli are naturally resistant to most nucleic acid inhibitors and to antibiotics (aminoglycosides and vancomycin) [12]. Antimicrobial resistance to other groups of antibiotics is different in different species of lactobacilli. High antimicrobial resistance to lincosamides, macrolides, and streptogramin was confirmed in lactobacilli (42–70%) [13,14]. At the same time, resistance to erythromycin, encoded by erm genes, which are often considered to be potentially transmissible genetic determinants, has recently been detected [15,16].

There are more than 30 *erm* genes [17]. The *ermB* gene, which encodes an rRNA methylase acting on the 23S ribosomal subunit, is very often detected in erythromycin-resistant lactobacilli. Other *erm* genes, such as *ermA*, *ermC* or *ermT*, have been confirmed in lactobacilli [18,19]. These *erm* genes can be found in transposons and plasmids and are propagated by conjugation mechanisms. Their nucleotide sequence and analysis of adjacent regions in the gene can give important information about their origin and the process of obtaining and transferring these determinants [20]. The transfer of some genes between *Lactobacillus* strains, and also from lactobacilli to Gram-positive bacteria and vice versa, has been found [21].

Detection of the phenotypic manifestation of antimicrobial resistance in lactobacilli alone is difficult, due to the absence of standards for antibiotic susceptibility testing. Existing limit values have been developed only for some antibiotics and the most commonly used probiotic species of lactobacilli [22]. In addition, the recently detected minimum inhibitor concentration (MIC) values for lactobacilli indicate acquired resistance, but it is not entirely clear whether the resistance in lactobacilli is caused by chromosomal mutations or by the acquisition of genetic factors. For this reason, it is still necessary to analyze mentioned bacteria with acquired resistance [23].

Based on these facts, isolates of the genus *Lactobacillus* will be identified in the study using matrix-assisted laser desorption/ionization mass spectrometry (MALDI-TOF-MS) and polymerase chain reaction (PCR) methods. Subsequently, antimicrobial resistance of *Lb. johnsonii* and *Lb. zeae* against selected antibiotics (ampicillin, clindamycin and erythromycin) will be detected by E-test and the broth microdilution method (BMM). At the same time, we want to confirm the presence of the *ermB* gene, which most often encodes erythromycin resistance in lactobacilli.

2. Materials and Methods

2.1. Isolation of Strains

In the study, samples of raw cows', sheep's, and goats' milk were used, which came from production farms located in eastern Slovakia. Samples of freshly milked milk were taken into sterile sample boxes (approximately 10 mL), according to the the principles of milk sampling STN EN ISO 6887-5 (2010) (Slovak Standards Institute, Bratislava, Slovakia) [24]. Fresh milk samples were tested during storage on the first, third, and seventh days. In order to research *Lactobacillus* sp., a total of 60 milk samples were analyzed. Of these, 20 samples in the number were cows', sheep's, and goats' milk, which were subjected to further examination.

Lactobacillus strains were isolated from the samples taken, according to the instructions of STN EN ISO 6887-1 (2017) (Slovak Standards Institute, Bratislava, Slovakia) [25]. From three successive dilutions, 0.1 mL of inoculum was inoculated by spreading on the surface of de Man, Rogosa, and Sharpe agar (MRS) selective diagnostic medium (Oxoid, Basingstoke, United Kingdom). Subsequent incubation was performed under anaerobic conditions at 37 °C for 24–72 h using AnaeroGen, which creates an anaerobic atmosphere (Oxoid, Basingstoke, United Kingdom).

For a more accurate identification of the genus *Lactobacillus* sp., suspected colonies were used, i.e., round cream–white convex colonies with a glossy surface of 2–5 mm. Selected colonies were inoculated into liquid BHI broth medium (Oxoid, Basingstoke, United Kingdom), using a sterile bacterial loop, and were incubated in anaerostat at 37 °C for 24–72 h under anaerobic conditions. After incubation, the propagated strains in liquid medium were used for genus and species identification by MALDI-TOF-MS and PCR.

2.2. Identification of Isolates

An extraction procedure using ethanol and formic acid was used to prepare samples for MALDI-TOF-MS identification. Analysis of the results was performed on an Ultraflex III instrument and Flex Analysis software, version 3.0. The results were evaluated using BioTyper software, version 1.1 (Bruker Daltonics, Massachusetts, United States), where the similarity between the mass spectra of the isolates and the reference mass spectrum of MALDI-TOF was expressed by scoring. A score greater than 2.30 represents a highly reliable identification at the species level; a score value between 2.00 and 2.29 means a highly reliable identification at the genus level, and a probable identification at the species level; a score value between 1.70 and 1.99 represents a reliable identification at the genus level; and a score value below 1.70 represents an unreliable identification [26]. The obtained identification results by MALDI-TOF-MS were confirmed by PCR method.

DNA from multiplied isolates was isolated using chelating agent Chelex 100 (Bio-Rad, Hertfordshire, United Kingdom), where 1.5 mL of bacterial culture was transferred to microtubes with 1 mL of sterile saline. The microtubes thus prepared were centrifuged at 10,000 g/10 min. The obtained sediment was resuspended in 200 mL of Chelex 100 chemical reagent and incubated at 95.5 °C/10 min. At the end of the incubation period, centrifugation was performed at 4 °C (13,000 g/3 min). The obtained supernatant was used as a source of DNA in PCR reactions.

Primers LbLMA (CTC AAA ACT AAA CAA AGT TCC) and R16 (ATG CGA TGC GAA TTT CTA ATT T) (AMPLIA s.r.o., Bratislava, Slovakia) [27] were used for genus identification of isolated strains by PCR method. The synthesized primers delimit the specific DNA sequence characteristic of the genus *Lactobacillus* spp., and where the size of the amplified fragment was 250 bp.

For species identification, we used ZeaI (TGT TTA GTT TTG AGG GGA CG) and ZeaII (CGT AAT GAG ATT TCA GTA GAT AAT ACA ACA) primers specific for *Lb. zeae* strains where the size of the amplified fragment was 185 bp. To identify *Lb. johnsonii*, JohSI (GAC CTT GCC TAG ATG ATT TTA) and 16SII (ACT ACC AGG GTA TCT AAT CC) primers were used, which delimited a specific sequence of 750 bp [11]. The Firepol Master Mix (Amplia s.r.o., Bratislava, Slovakia) was used in the PCR reactions.

Initiation denaturation was at 95 °C/3 min, followed by 30 amplification cycles (denaturation at 95 °C for 20 s; annealing at 55 °C/30 s for LbLMA/R16, and at 57 °C/30 s for ZeaI/ZeaII and JohSI/16SII; extension at 72 °C/2 min) was used to amplify specific sequences. The last cycle was followed by a final extension at 72 °C/10 min. Reference strains—*Lb. zeae* CCM 7069 and *Lb. johnsonii* CCM 2935 and *Lb. paracasei* CCM 4649 (Czech Collection of Microorganisms, Brno, Czech Republic)—were used to verify the specificity of the PCR reaction. The amplified PCR product in an amount of 5 µL was analyzed on a 1.5% agarose gel in Tris-Borate-EDTA (TBE) solution. We added Goldview Nucleic (Beijing SBS Genetech, Beijing, China) to the agarose gels for DNA visualization. Electrophoresis was performed for 1 h at 120 V. Individual PCR fragments were visualized using a Mini Bis Pro reader (DNR Bio-Imaging systems Ltd., Neve Yamin, Israel). The sizes of the resulting PCR products were determined based on their mobility in agarose gels compared to a 100 bp standard (Sigma-Aldrich, United States).

The identity of the PCR products with the selected primers was confirmed by a commercial company (GATC Biotech AG, Cologne, Germany). The DNA sequences obtained from strains were searched for homology to those available at the GenBank–EMBL (The European Molecular Biology Laboratory) database using the BLAST program (NCBI software package).

2.3. Antimicrobial Resistance

The phenotypic manifestation of antimicrobial resistance in strains of *Lactobacillus* sp. against ampicillin (AMP), erythromycin (ERY), and clindamycin (CLI) was determined using a semi-quantitative E-test method [28]. To determine antibiotic susceptibility by E-test, an inoculum adjusted to a standard density of 0.5 McF° (degree of McFarland's turbidity standard) was inoculated onto the surface of Müller–Hinton agar medium enriched with 10% MRS agar (Oxford, United

Kingdom). After soaking the inoculum, a test strip with a well-defined antibiotic content was applied sterile to the inoculated surface of the agar medium. The test plates thus prepared were incubated at 37 °C for 18–24 h. After the determined incubation, a teardrop-shaped zone of inhibition (drops) formed on the surface of the Petri dishes. The minimum inhibitor concentration (MIC) value was determined according to the manufacturer´s instructions, so that the resulting MIC value corresponded to the concentration of antibiotics on the strip where the edges of the inhibition zone converged. The E-test was read according to the manufacturer´s instructions, which specified reading at the point of complete inhibition of all growth.

Subsequently, antimicrobial resistance was determined using the broth microdilution method (BMM) [28]. Mueller–Hinton broth plates supplemented with lysed horse blood (Oxoid, Basingstoke, United Kingdom) were used for testing. The test plates contained concentrations of 0.125, 0.250, 0.500, 1.000, 2.000, 4.000, 8.000, 16.000, and 32.000 mg/L of each tested antibiotic. *Streptococcus pneumoniae* CCM 4501 (Czech collection of microorganisms, Brno, Czech Republic) was used as a reference strain. After incubation, the lowest concentrations of antibiotics that inhibited the visible growth of the test strains were determined. The results were evaluated according to document CLSI (Clinical laboratory Standards Institute, Wayne, Pennsylvania, US) [28].

After evaluating the phenotypic properties of antimicrobial resistance, the genetic determinant of erythromycin resistance of the *ermB* gene was detected using primers ermB2-F (GAAAAGGTACTCAACCAAATA) and ermB2-R (AGTAACGGTACTTAAATTGTTTAC), as well as the FIREpol Master Mix (Amplia s.r.o., Slovakia) [29]. The PCR reaction was performed as for genus and species identification of bacterial isolates, except for annealing, where the temperature was adjusted to 59 °C. The final PCR product was 639 bp in size. DNA sequences obtained from strains were searched for homology to those available from the GenBank–EMBL database using the BLAST program (NCBI software package). *Staphylococcus aureus* CCM 4223 showing the presence of the *ermB* gene was used as a reference strain [30].

2.4. Statistical Analyses

For statistical analyses, one-way analysis of variance (ANOVA) was used, along with a Tukey test for multiple comparison of means, with a confidence interval set at 95%, which was conducted with statistics software GraphPad Prism 8.3.0.538 (GraphPad Software, San Diego, CA, United States). The various types of milk were set as main factor.

3. Results

The occurrence of lactobacili in raw milk is well-known. They play an important role in the gastrointestinal tract of the consumer and in the production of fermented dairy products. Several types of lactobacili are present in individual kinds of milk. This study points on the possible occurrence of species *Lb. johnsonii* and *Lb. zeae* in raw milk and not only in fermented dairy products and cheeses.

During the cultivation of milk samples during the first, third, and seventh days, the lowest number of lactobacilli colonies per day was recorded during the seventh day, at 3.7 ± 0.1 log CFU/mL in cows' milk and 1.8 ± 0.1 log CFU/mL in goats' milk. The highest number of lactobacilli colonies in goats' milk (2.0 ± 0.1 log CFU/mL) was measured on the first day of measurement. In cows' milk, the number of colonies during the first and third days was the same (3.8 ± 0.1 log CFU/mL). In sheep's milk, the number of colonies counted during the first, third, and seventh days did not change, and remained the same at 3.2 ± 0.1 log CFU/mL (Table 1).

Table 1. Number of lactobacilli colonies (log CFU/mL) obtained by culture microbiological examination of milk samples using de Man, Rogosa, and Sharpe (MRS) agar medium (mean ± SD).

Kind of Milk	Day 1	Day 3	Day 7
Cows' milk	3.8 ± 0.1 [a;1]	3.8 ± 0.1 [a;1]	3.7 ± 0.1 [a;1]
Sheep´s milk	3.2 ± 0.1 [a;2]	3.2 ± 0.1 [a;2]	3.2 ± 0.1 [a;2]
Goats' milk	2.0 ± 0.1 [a;3]	1.9 ± 0.1 [ab;3]	1.8 ± 0.1 [b;3]

[1, 2, 3] Within the columns, values with different numbers are significantly different at $p < 0.05$. [a, b] Within the row, values with different letters are significantly different at $p < 0.05$.

In our study, a total of 60 individual milk samples were examined, of which one-third was represented by raw cows' milk, one-third by raw sheep's milk, and one-third by raw goats' milk. Table 1 shows the average values numbers of lactobacilli colonies (log CFU/mL) from all analyzed milk samples during the tested period. Microbial quality parameters represented by numbers of lactobacilli colonies (log CFU/mL) in different types of milk were changed during storage (Table 1). There was a statistically significant change ($p < 0.05$) in the goats' milk in the number of lactobacilli between the first day (2.0 ± 0.1 log CFU/mL) and the seventh day (1.8 ± 0.1 log CFU/mL) of milk storage. No statistically significant change in the number of lactobacilli in cows' and sheep's milk was detected during the storage. However, on the first, third, and seventh measured days of the study, the number of lactobacilli colonies showed a statistically significant difference ($p < 0.001$) between all types of tested milk (cows', sheep's, and goats').

By microbiological examination of the culture samples of individual types of raw milk (cows', sheep's, and goats' milk), a total of 300 strains were isolated using the selective diagnostic medium MRS agar, which formed typical colonies according to their phenotypic growth characteristics.

For genus and species identification of individual isolated strains from all types of milk, the MALDI-TOF-MS method was used, which identified 252 isolates from 300 strains as *Lactobacillus* sp. with score values of 1.658–2.258. Subsequently, for further identification we selected only strains that were identified as *Lb. johnsonii* (26 isolates; 10.3%) and *Lb. zeae* (19 isolates; 7.5%) (Table 2). The score value ranged from 1.698 to 2.176 with *Lb. johnsonii* and from 1.734 to 2.246 for *Lb. zeae*. The score value of the isolates was below 2.300, which means that the identification of the isolates at the species level was not sufficiently reliable; therefore, the PCR method was used to confirm the results obtained by MALDI-TOF-MS (Table 2).

Table 2. The number of identified strains of *Lactobacillus* sp. and *Lb. johnsonii* and *Lb. zeae* species in milk samples.

		Lactobacillus sp.	*Lb. johnsonii*	*Lb. zeae*
Cows' milk	MALDI-TOF-MS	131	10	8
	PCR	128	10	8
Sheep's milk	MALDI-TOF-MS	80	10	5
	PCR	77	7	5
Goats' milk	MALDI-TOF-MS	41	6	6
	PCR	40	6	5
Σ	MALDI-TOF-MS	252	26	19
	PCR	245	23	18

MALDI-TOF-MS: matrix-assisted laser desorption/ionization mass spectrometry; PCR: polymerase chain reaction; Σ: summary.

Subsequently, the molecular PCR method was used for accurate identification at the genus and species level [27].

In Figure 1 a PCR product of 250 bp in length was detected using specific primers for the genus *Lactobacillus*. Based on the visualized fragments and their subsequent sequencing, the genus *Lactobacillus* sp. confirmed in 245 strains isolated from samples of all types of raw milk. The species identification of isolates was performed by using specific synthesized primers [15]. *Lb. johnsonii* (Figure 2) and *Lb. zeae* (Figure 3) have been identified.

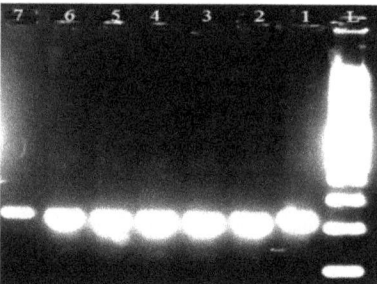

Figure 1. Identification of genus *Lactobacillus* sp. L: 100 bp ladder standard; lines 1, 2, 3, and 4: isolates of *Lactobacillius* sp. (250 bp); line 5: *Lb. johnsonii* reference strain CCM 2935; line 6: *Lb. zeae* reference strain CCM 7069; line 7: *Lb. paracasei* reference strain CCM 4649.

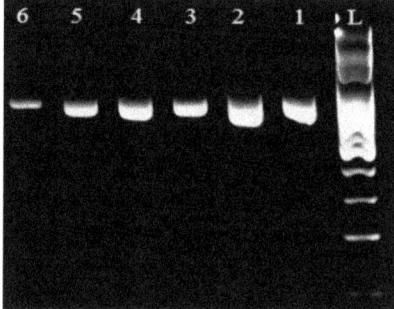

Figure 2. Identification of genus *Lb. johnsonii*. L: 100 bp ladder standard; lines 1, 2, 3, 4, and 5: *Lb. johnsonii* isolates (750 bp); line 6: *Lb. johnsonii* reference strain CCM 2935.

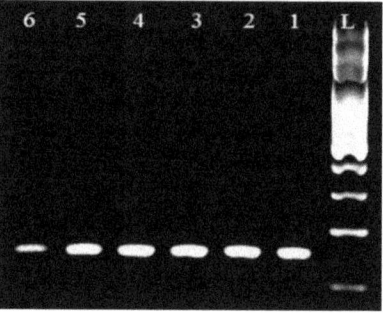

Figure 3. Identification of genus *Lb. zeae*. L: 100 bp standard; line 1: *Lb. zeae* reference strain CCM 7069 (750 bp); lines 2, 3, 4, and 5: *Lb. zeae* isolates.

When comparing the representation of *Lactobacillus* sp. for various types of milk, the highest incidence of this genus, confirmed by PCR, was in cows' raw milk (128 isolates), and the lowest was in goats' raw milk (40 isolates). From strains of the genus *Lactobacillus* sp., the species *Lb. johnsonii* was, among the selected samples of raw milk, the most represented in goats' milk (15.0%) and the least in cows' milk (7.8%). *Lb. zeae* was also predominantly isolated from goats' milk (12.5%), while in sheep's (6.5%) and cows' milk (6.3%) it had a similar proportion of isolates. These results correspond to the results of the MALDI-TOF-MS identification, despite that the results of the identification of both methods differing in some isolates. Conflicting identification occurred in three *Lb. johnsonii* strains and one *Lb. zeae* strain. However, these isolates showed a low score value between 1.698–1.792 when identified, indicating the reliability of identification only at the genus level.

In the next part of the study, only strains identified as *Lb. johnsonii* (23 isolates) and *Lb. zeae* (18 isolates) by MALDI-TOF-MS and PCR were used to determine antimicrobial resistance.

When determining susceptibility by E-test, the MIC for each identified antibiotic tested was detected in the range of 0.125–16.000 µg/mL for species-identified isolates (41 isolates) (Table 3). As there are no uniform standards for determining antimicrobial resistance in the lactobacilli species we tested, we proceeded to evaluate the obtained MIC values [28]. Strains whose MIC for ampicillin was >8 µg/mL and for erythromycim was ≥8 µg/mL were considered resistant. For clindamycin, resistant strains were considered to be those with an MIC ≥ 2 µg/mL. Based on these criteria, 7.3% of lactobacilli strains were evaluated as ampicillin-resistant, 14.7% of isolates as erythromycin-resistant, and 4.9% of isolates as clindamycin-resistant. The genus *Lb. johnsonii* had the highest resistance to erythromycin (34.8%), but no strain was resistant to clindamycin. The genus *Lb. zeae* also showed the greatest resistance to erythromycin (33.3%), and this species was also confirmed to be resistant to clindamycin (Table 3).

Table 3. MIC determination of test isolates by E-test.

Strains	ATB	MIC µg/mL											
		0.125	0.19	0.25	0.5	0.75	1	1.5	2	3	4	8	12	16	32
Lb. johnsonii (n = 23)	AMP	2	1	4	6	1	1			3	2	1		1		1
	ERY	4		1	7	1			2			4	2	2	
	CLI			8	11		4								
Lb. zeae (n = 18)	AMP	2	2	6	2	3	1					1	1		
	ERY	3		5	1	1			2			2	1	3	
	CLI	9	1	4		1	1		1	1					

MIC: minimal inhibitory concentration; AMP: ampicillin; ERY: erythromycin; CLI: clindamycin; n: number of isolates. Only antibiotic concentrations at which the MIC was recorded for at least one strain are shown in the table.

As the determination of susceptibility to individual antibiotics in lactobacilli is difficult to test, we also proceeded with antimicrobial resistance testing using the broth microdilution method (BMM).

As shown in Table 4, resistant strains were detected for all antibiotics tested. The highest number of resistant strains was, similarly to the E-test, confirmed against erythromycin (14.7%), and the smallest against clindamycin (7.3%). Minor discrepancies in the results of both methods occurred in the detection of susceptibility to ampicillin and clindamycin.

Table 4. MIC determination of *Lb. johnsonii* and *Lb. zeae* isolates using the broth dilution method.

	Strains	Lb. johnsonii			Lb. zeae		
	Antibiotic	AMP	ERY	CLI	AMP	ERY	CLI
MIC µg/mL	0.125	2	3	1	4	3	10
	0.250	5	2	8	6	5	4
	0.500	7	8	10	5	2	1
	1.000	1		3	1		1
	2.000	5	2	1		2	1
	4.000	1					1
	8.000		6			2	
	16.000	1	2		2	4	
	32.000	1					

MIC-minimal inhibitory concentration; AMP: ampicillin; ERY: erythromycin; CLI: clindamycin. Gray color represents breakpoint that categorizes lactobacilli as "resistant".

When determining the susceptibility to ampicillin, one strain of *Lb. zeae* was marked as susceptible based on the determined MIC (8 µg/mL) by E-test, but with the BMM method, the MIC was found to be 16 µg/mL, and therefore was marked as resistant. One *Lb. johnsonii* strain was evaluated as intermediate sensitive by E-test (MIC was 1.0 µg/mL). However, it was assessed as resistant by BMM, as the MIC was determined to be 2.0 µg/mL.

In one *Lb. johnsonii* isolate, resistance to two antibiotics was confirmed simultaneously by both methods; namely, it was resistance to ampicillin and erythromycin. When comparing the resistance of tested lactobacilli from the different types of examined milk, most resistant strains occurred in lactobacilli isolated from cows' milk (Figure 4).

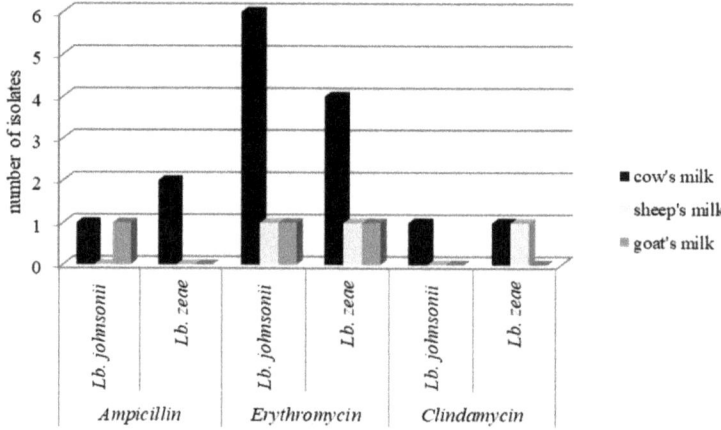

Figure 4. Number of resistant strains in each type of milk.

As erythromycin resistance predominated in the determination of the phenotypic manifestation of antimicrobial resistance, we proceeded to detect the *ermB* gene, which according to previous studies, is often detected in erythromycin-resistant lactobacilli.

The PCR method confirmed the presence of the *ermB* gene in 7 of 41 isolates of species-identified lactobacilli (Figure 5), namely the five strains of *Lb. johnsonii* (four isolates of cows' milk and one isolate of goats' milk) and two strains of *Lb. zeae* (one isolate of cows' milk and one isolate of sheep's milk). Isolates in which the presence of the *ermB* gene was confirmed had a phenotypic manifestation of erythromycin resistance.

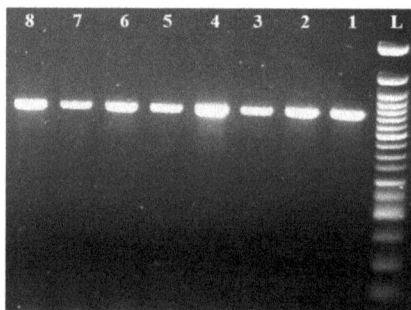

Figure 5. Identification of the *ermB* gene in *Lactobacillus* sp. L: 50 bp standard; line 1: *Staphylococcus aureus* reference strain CCM 4223 (639 bp); lines 2–3: isolates of *Lb. zeae* with *ermB* gene; lines 4–8: isolates of *Lb. johnsonii* with *ermB* gene.

4. Discussion

Lactobacilli form a significant microbial population of raw milk are widely present in various fermented dairy products. Their presence in several types of raw milk was also confirmed in this study, where the number of bacteria of the genus *Lactobacillus* sp. was in fresh cows' milk (3.8 ± 0.1 log CFU/mL), sheep's milk (3.2 ± 0.1 log CFU/mL), and goats' milk (2.0 ± 0.1 log CFU/mL). The presence of lactobacilli in raw milk has been confirmed by several studies, including Vataščinová et al., where in 23 geographical areas of Eastern Slovakia, 43 strains have been identified as *Lactobacillus* sp. [31]. However, the high nutrient content of raw milk during storage makes it a suitable medium for a large number of other microorganisms, such as *C. perfringens*, *S. aureus*, *E. coli*, *L. monocytogenes*, *Salmonella* spp., *Bacillus cereus*, *Streptococcus* sp., etc., which develop rapidly in it and cause its deterioration [32].

This leads to a decrease in quality due to changes in its organoleptic, technological, and other properties. At the same time, the microflora of lactobacilli is suppressed, and undesirable microorganisms develop in samples of stored raw milk [33]. The suppression of lactobacilli microflora during storage of all types of milk is also indicated by the results of this study. In addition, differences in lactobacilli counts were observed between milk species. These differences are given by the differential chemical composition of cows', sheep's, and goats milk, as well as geographical areas [34]. Many studies have addressed the species identification of lactobacilli, but few studies indicate the detection of *Lb. johnsonii* and *Lb. zeae* species from various types of raw milk [34]. *Lb. zeae* is described as a closely related species of *Lb. casei* [10]. A group of species *Lb. casei* includes *Lb. casei*, *Lb. paracasei* subsp. *Paracasei*, *Lb. paracasei* subsp. *Tolerans*, *Lb. rhamnosus*, and *Lb. zeae*. The first three species are commonly isolated from milk and dairy products, and play an important role in human and animal nutrition as a probiotic [35]. *Lb. johnsonii*, in turn, is largely involved in the colonization of the gastrointestinal tract and its functional properties related to its ability to adhere to the intestinal mucosa, resist bile and acids, or colonize the intestines and produce bacteriocin [36]. Due to the positive properties and low uptake in fresh milk, another part of this study focused on the detection of the above-mentioned types of lactobacilli.

Identification was performed by MALDI-TOF-MS and PCR method. Using MALDI-TOF-MS, from 300 isolated strains, 252 isolates were identified as *Lactobacillus* sp. with the score value 1658–2258. A total of 26 isolates were confirmed as *Lb. johnsonii* species, and 19 isolates as *Lb. zeae*. The score value ranged from 1.698 to 2.176 for *Lb. johnsonii*, and from 1.734 to 2.246 for species *Lb. zeae*. Dec et al. identified four species of lactobacilli—*Lb. casei*, *Lb. johnsonii*, *Lb. kitasatonis*, and *Lb. zeae*—in foods of animal origin, but with low score values comparable to our study. He also described the lack of discriminatory ability to distinguish closely related species, such as *Lb. johnsonii*, *Lb. gasseri*, *Lb. crispatus*, *Lb. ultunensis*, *Lb. oris*, and *Lb. antri* by MALDI-TOF-MS [14].

In a presented study, there was no score value for confirmation of a species more than 2.30. We approached the detection using PCR method, which is considered to be one of the foundation stones of modern microbial taxonomy [26].

PCR is a standard method for identifying bacteria and determining microbial diversity, and is widely applied to the *Lactobacillus* genus, which is the result of the high specificity of the gene sequence 16s rDNA for each bacterial species [37]. Using specific primers, we verified the presence of the genus *Lactobacillus* sp. in 245 isolated strains [27]. Subsequent species-level identification detected a species-specific PCR product *Lb. zeae* (7.5%) in 19 isolates, and *Lb. johnsonii* in 26 isolates (representing 10.3% of identified lactobacilli) [11]. The other studies reported that of the 47 strains of *Lactobacillus* sp. isolated from different media, 16 strains were identified as *Lb. johnsonii* by multiplex PCR [36]. Delaveane et al. research antifungal strains of *Lactobacillus* sp. (including *Lb. zeae*) previously isolated from cows' and goats' milk. All showed different acidification and growth capacities, which makes *Lb. zeae* a potential candidate for yogurt biopreservation [38].

Microorganism resistance to antibiotics is a current global problem. A major role in the spread of lactobacillus resistance in the food chain is the ill-considered choice of antibiotics in the treatment of food animals [39]. The new findings also point to the presence of resistant strains in probiotic bacteria (including the genus *Lactobacillus*), the use of which has a positive effect on the intestinal microflora in humans and animals [40,41]. Antibiotic resistance of probiotic bacteria has recently been perceived as a risk to the consumer. Bacteria belonging to the group of probiotics show a so-called natural resistance to metronidazole, colistin, and vancomycin [42].

In our study, the antimicrobial resistance was detected by two methods: E-test and broth microdilution method to ampicillin, clindamycin, and, to a greater extent, erythromycin (*Lb. johnsonii* = 34.8% and *Lb. zeae* = 33.3%). The highest agreement when comparing the MIC determination by E-test and BMM was detected for erythromycin. A lower level of agreement was detected for ampicillin and clindamycin, where some isolates showed lower MICs in the E-test. Similarly, Mayrhofer et al. detected the levels of agreement between these methods that were high for the antimicrobial agents ampicillin, gentamicin, streptomycin, and vancomycin (90%) [43]. Lower levels of agreement were obtained for clindamycin (71%), erythromycin (80%), and especially tetracycline (34%). In general, lower MICs of ampicillin, clindamycin, erythromycin, and streptomycin were obtained by E-test. Discrepancies in the determination of MIC by the E-test and BMM method have also been pointed out by Kushiro et al. for only 5% of cases with three antimicrobials (tetracycline, rifampicin, and kanamycin), and a more than four-fold difference between the two methods has been observed [44]. The biggest differences were shown with *Lb. delbrueckii* for rifampicin. The BMM method also confirmed the resistance of several antibiotics in lactobacilli [14].

Resistance to at least three groups of antimicrobials was observed in 64.5% of lactobacilli, and 43.5% of isolates showed cross-resistance between erythromycin and lincomycin. Resistance to streptomycin and gentamicin was recorded simultaneously for 6% of isolates. Acquired resistance was observed for erythromycin, lincomycin, and tetracycline. Sharma et al. detected multiresistance and polyresistance in lactobacilli strains, as well as other lactobacilli. Multiple resistance to the most commonly used antibiotics, such as norfloxacin, teicoplanin, cefepime, and amikacin, has been confirmed in most isolates. Lactobacilli has shown low levels of resistance to, for example, ampicillin, cefaclor, gentamicin, oxacillin, tetracycline, and novobiocin [45]. Recently, erythromycin resistance has also been increasingly detected in lactobacilli. Major genes responsible for erythromycin resistance are *erm* (*A*), *erm*(*C*), *erm*(*T*), and *erm*(*B*), which encode rRNA methylase acting on the 23 S subunit, which is predominate in *Lactobacillus* genus [45–47]. This is also confirmed by our study, where this gene was confirmed in 17% of lactobacilli isolates isolated from raw milk. The phenotypic manifestation of antimicrobial resistance of the tested lactobacilli was associated with the presence of the *ermB* gene. Drago et al. also confirmed erythromycin resistance in more than one-third of 40 lactobacillus isolates. Again, macrolide resistance was mostly associated with the presence of the *ermB* gene [48].

This study confirmed the presence of resistant strains *Lb. zeae* and *Lb. johnsonii* in various types of raw milk. At the same time, the *ermB* gene, which is responsible for encoding erythromycin resistance, was detected in these strains. The presence of these resistant strains, even in raw milk, indicates an increased risk of the possibility of the spread of resistance across the food chain.

Author Contributions: Conceptualization, J.V.; methodology, J.V. and I.R.; software, M.K.; formal analysis, E.D. and S.M.; investigation and data curation, J.V., M.K., and J.M.; writing—original draft preparation, J.V.; writing—review and editing, I.R. and E.D.; supervision, I.R. and J.V.; project administration and funding acquisition, J.M. and I.R. All authors have read and agreed to the published version of the manuscript.

Funding: This work was supported by the following grants: APVV-19-0234, "Development of probiotic preparation based on autochthonous lactobacilli for salmonids intended to improve fish health and production of quality food"; and KEGA 007UVLF-4/2020, "Innovation of milk and milk products hygiene and technology education" at the University of Veterinary Medicine and Pharmacy in Košice.

Conflicts of Interest: The authors declare no conflict of interest.

References

1. Zhang, H.; Cai, Y. *Lactic Acid Bacteria: Fundamentals and Practice*; Springer: Berlin/Heidelberg, Germany, 2014; p. 535. ISBN 978-94-017-8841-0.

2. Mozzi, F.; Raya, R.R.; Vignolo, G.M.; Love, J.C. *Biotechnology of Lactic Acid Bacteria: Novel Applications*; John Wiley and Sons: Hoboken, NJ, USA, 2010; p. 352. ISBN 978-0-8138-1583-1.
3. Baruzzi, F.; Poltronieri, P.; Quero, G.M.; Morea, M.; Morelli, L. An in vitro protocol for direct isolation of potential probiotic Lactobacilli from raw bovine milk and traditional fermented milks. *Appl. Microbiol. Biotechnol.* **2011**, *90*, 331–342. [CrossRef]
4. Košta, M.; Slottová, A.; Dronćovský, M.; Klapáčová, L.; Kmeť, V.; Bujňáková, D.; Lauková, A.; Grief, G.; Griefová, M.; Tomáška, M. Characterisation of Lactobacilli from ewe's and goat's milk for their further processing re-utilisation. *Potravin. Slovak J. Food Sci.* **2014**, *8*, 130–134.
5. Tomáška, M.; Dronćovský, M.; Klapáčová, L.; Slottová, A.; Košta, M. Potential probiotic properties of Lactobacilli isolated from goat´s milk. *Potravin. Slovak J. Food Sci.* **2015**, *9*, 66–71. [CrossRef]
6. Vukotić, G.; Strahinić, I.; Begović, J.; Lukić, J.; Kojić, M.; Fira, D. Survey on proteolytic activity and diversity of proteinase genes in mesophilic lactobacilli. *Microbiology* **2016**, *85*, 33–41. [CrossRef]
7. Lim, S.D.; Kim, K.S.; Do, J.R. Physiological characteristics and ACE inhibitory activity of *Lactobacillus zeae* RMK354 isolated from raw milk. *Korean. J. Food Sci. Anl. Resour.* **2008**, *28*, 587–595. [CrossRef]
8. Henri-Dubernet, S.; Desmasures, N.; Gueguen, M. Diversity and dynamics of lactobacilli populations during ripening of RDO Camembert cheese. *Can. J. Microbiol.* **2008**, *54*, 218–228. [CrossRef] [PubMed]
9. Salyers, A.A.; Shoemaker, N.B.; Stevens, A.M.; Li, L.Y. Conjugative transposons: An unusual and diverse set of integrated gene transfer elements. *Microbiol. Rev.* **1995**, *59*, 579–590. [CrossRef] [PubMed]
10. Eid, R.; El Jakee, J.; Rashidy, A.; Asfour, H.; Omara, S.; Kandil, M.M.I.; Mahmood, Z.; Hahne, J.; Seida, A.A. Potential antimicrobial activities of probiotic Lactobacillus strains isolated from raw milk. *J. Prob. Health* **2016**, *4*. [CrossRef]
11. Walter, J.; Tannock, G.W.; Tilasala-Timisjarvi, A.; Rodtong, S.; Loach, D.M.; Munro, K.; Alatossava, T. Detection and Identification of Gastrointestinal Lactobacillus Species by Using Denaturing Gradient Gel Electrophoresis and Species-Specific PCR Primers. *Appl. Environ. Microbiol.* **2000**, *66*, 297–303. [CrossRef]
12. Gueimonde, M.; Sánchez, B.; de los Reyes-Gavilán, C.G.; Margolles, A. Antibiotic resistance in probiotic bacteria. *Front. Microbiol.* **2013**, *4*, 202. [CrossRef]
13. Klare, I.; Konstabel, C.; Müller-Bertling, S.; Reissbrodt, R.; Huys, G.; Vancanneyt, M.; Witte, W. Evaluation of new broth media for microdilution antibiotic susceptibility testing of lactobacilli, pediococci, lactococci, and bifidobacteria. *Appl. Environ. Microbiol.* **2005**, *71*, 8982–8986. [CrossRef] [PubMed]
14. Dec, M.; Nowaczek, A.; Stępień-Pyśniak, D.; Wawrzykowski, J.; Urban-Chmiel, R. Identification and antibiotic susceptibility of lactobacilli isolated from turkeys. *BMC Microbiol.* **2018**, *18*, 168. [CrossRef]
15. Roberts, M.C. Update on acquired tetracycline resistance genes. *FEMS Microbiol. Lett.* **2005**, *245*, 195–203. [CrossRef] [PubMed]
16. Roberts, M.C. Update on macrolide-lincosamide-streptogramin, ketolide, and oxazolidinone resistance genes. *FEMS Microbiol. Lett.* **2008**, *282*, 147–159. [CrossRef] [PubMed]
17. Roberts, M.C.; Sutcliffe, J.; Courvalin, P.; Jensen, L.B.; Rood, J.; Seppala, H. Nomenclature for macrolide and macrolide-lincosamide-streptogramin B resistance determinants. *Antimicrob. Agents Chemother.* **1999**, *43*, 2823–2830. [CrossRef] [PubMed]
18. Van Hoek, A.H.A.M.; Margolles, A.; Damig, K.J.; Korhonen, J.M.; ZyckaKrzesinka, J.; Bardowsky, J.; Danielsen, M.; Huys, G.; Morelli, L.; Aarts, H.J.M. Molecular assessment of erythromycin and tetracycline resistance genes in lactic acid bacteria and bifidobacteria and their relation to the phenotypic resistance. *Int. J. Probiotics Prebiotics* **2008**, *3*, 271–280.
19. Mayrhofer, S.; van Hoek, A.H.; Mair, C.; Huys, G.; Aarts, H.J.; Kneifel, W.; Domig, K.J. Antibiotic susceptibility of members of the Lactobacillus acidophilus group using broth microdilution and molecular identification of their resistance determinants. *Int. J. Food Microbiol.* **2010**, *144*, 81–87. [CrossRef]
20. Aquilanti, L.; Garofalo, C.; Osimani, A.; Silvestri, G.; Vignaroli, C.; Clementi, F. Isolation and molecular characterization of antibiotic-resistant lactic acid bacteria from poultry and swine meat products. *J. Food Prot.* **2007**, *70*, 557–565. [CrossRef]
21. Tannock, G.W.; Luchansky, J.B.; Miller, L.; Connell, H.; Thode-Andersen, S.; Mercer, A.A.; Klaenhammer, T.R. Molecular characterization of a plasmid-borne (pGT633) erythromycin resistance determinant (ermGT) from Lactobacillus reuteri 100–63. *Plasmid* **1994**, *31*, 60–71. [CrossRef]

22. EFSA. Technical guidance prepared by the panel on additives and Products or substances used in animal feed (FEEDAP) on the update of the criteria used in the assessment of bacterial resistance to antibiotics of human or veterinary importance (question no. EFSA-Q-2008-004). *EFSA J.* **2008**, *732*, 1–15.
23. Cauwerts, K.; Pasmans, F.; Devriese, L.A.; Martel, A.; Haesebrouck, F.; Decostere, A. Cloacal Lactobacillus isolates from broilers show high prevalence of resistance towards macrolide and lincosamide antibiotics. *Avian Pathol.* **2006**, *35*, 160–164. [CrossRef] [PubMed]
24. STN EN ISO 6887-5. *Microbiology of Food and Animal Feeding Stuffs. Preparation of Test Samples, Initial Suspension and Decimal Dilutions for Microbiological Examination. Part 5: Specific Rules for the Preparation of Milk and Milk Products (ISO 6887-5:2010)*; Slovak Standards Institute: Bratislava, Slovak, 2010.
25. STN EN ISO 6887-1. *Microbiology of the Food Chain-Preparation of Test Samples, Initial Suspension and Decimal Dilutions for Microbiological Examination-Part 1: General Rules for the Preparation of the Initial Suspension and Decimal Dilutions (ISO 6887-1:2017)*; Slovak Standards Institute: Bratislava, Slovak, 2017.
26. Bruker Daltonics. *MALDI Biotyper 2.0. Software for Microorganism Identification and Classification User Manual*; Bruker Corporation: Billerica, MA, USA, 2008.
27. Dubernet, S.; Desmasures, N.; Guéguen, M.A. PCR-based method for identification of Lactobacilli at the genus level. *FEMS Microbiol. Lett.* **2002**, *214*, 271–275. [CrossRef] [PubMed]
28. CLSI document M–45. *Methods for Antimicrobial Dilution and Disk Susceptibility Testing of Infrequently Isolated or Fastidious Bacteria*; Clinical and Laboratory Standards Institute: Wayne, PA, USA, 2015.
29. Sutcliffe, J.; Grebe, T.; Tait-Kamradt, A.; Wondrack, L. Detection of erythromycin-resistant determinants by PCR. *Antimicrob. Agents Chemother.* **1996**, *40*, 2562–2566. [CrossRef]
30. Anisimova, E.; Yarullina, D. Characterization of erythromycin and tetracycline resistance in Lactobacillus fermentum strains. *Int. J. Microbiol.* **2018**. [CrossRef] [PubMed]
31. Vataščinová, T.; Pipová, M.; Fraqueza, M.J.R.; Mala, P.; Dudriková, E.; Drážovská, M.; Lauková, A. Antimicrobial potential of Lactobacillus plantarum strains isolated from Slovak raw sheep milk cheeses. *J. Dairy Sci.* **2019**, *103*, 6900–6903. [CrossRef] [PubMed]
32. Tan, S.F.; Chin, N.L.; Tee, T.P.; Chooi, S.K. Physico-Chemical Changes, Microbiological Properties, and Storage Shelf Life of Cow and Goat Milk from Industrial High-Pressure Processing. *Processes* **2020**, *8*, 697. [CrossRef]
33. Ebringer, L.; Soják, L. Mlieko ako multifunkčná potravina. *Interná Med.* **2007**, *7–8*, 423–427.
34. Mahdavi, S.; Isazadeh, A.; Azimian, S.H.; Bonab, N.M.; Shekar, F.; Asgharian, A. Isolation of Lactobacillus Species from Domestic Dairy Products of Mahabad City. *Int. J. Infect.* **2018**, *5*, 62152. [CrossRef]
35. Pantoflickova, D.; Corthésy-Theulaz, I.; Stolte, M.; Isler, P.; Rochat, F.; Enslen, M.; Blum, A.L. Favourable effect of regular intake of fermented milk containing Lactobacillus johnsonii on Helicobacter pylori associated gastritis. *Aliment. Pharmacol. Ther.* **2003**, *18*, 805–813. [CrossRef]
36. Ventura, M.; Zink, R. Specific identification and molecular typing analysis of Lactobacillus johnsonii by using PCR-based methods and pulsed-field gel electrophoresis. *FEMS Microbiol. Lett.* **2002**, *17*, 141–154. [CrossRef]
37. Nemska, V.; Lazarova, N.; Georgieva, N.; Danova, S. Lactobacillus spp. From traditional Bulgarian dairy products. *J. Chem. Technol. Met.* **2016**, *51*, 693–704.
38. Delavenne, E.; Ismail, R.; Pawtowski, A.; Mounier, J.; Barbier, G.; Le Blay, G. Assessment of lactobacilli strains as yogurt bioprotective cultures. *Food Control.* **2013**, *30*, 206–213. [CrossRef]
39. Collingnon, P. Antibiotic resistance: Are we all doomed. *Intern. Med. J.* **2015**, *45*, 1109–1115. [CrossRef] [PubMed]
40. Borriello, S.P.; Hammes, W.P.; Holzapfel, W.; Marteau, P.; Schrezenmeir, J.; Vaara, M.; Valtonen, V. Safety of probiotics that contain lactobacilli or bifidobacteria. *Clin. Infect. Dis.* **2003**, *36*, 775–780. [CrossRef] [PubMed]
41. Rowland, I.; Capurso, L.; Collins, K.; Cummings, J.; Delzenne, N.; Goulet, O.; Guarner, F.; Marteau, P.; Meier, R. Current level of consensus on probiotic science. Report of an expert meeting London 23 November 2009. *Gut Microbes* **2010**, *1*, 436–439. [CrossRef] [PubMed]
42. Adekunle, O. Effect of Probiotics in the Mitigation of *Clostridium difficile* Associated Disease. Diploma Thesis, Georgia State University, Atlanta, GA, USA, 2015.
43. Mayrhofer, S.; Domig, K.J.; Mair, C.; Zitz, U.; Huys, G.; Kneifel, W. Comparison of Broth Microdilution, Etest, and Agar Disk Diffusion Methods for Antimicrobial Susceptibility Testing of Lactobacillus acidophilus Group Members. *Appl. Environ. Microbiol.* **2008**, *12*, 3745–3748. [CrossRef] [PubMed]

44. Kushiro, A.; Chervaux, C.; Cools-Portier, S.; Perony, A.; Legrain-Raspaud, S.; Obis, D.; Onoue, M.; van de Moer, A. Antimicrobial susceptibility testing of lactic acid bacteria and bifidobacteria by broth microdilution method and Etest. *Int. J. Food Microbiol.* **2009**, *132*, 54–58. [CrossRef]
45. Sharma, P.; Tomar, S.; Sangwan, V.; Goswami, P.; Singh, R. Antibiotic Resistance of Lactobacillus sp. isolated from commercial probiotic preparations. *J. Food Saf.* **2016**, *36*, 38–51. [CrossRef]
46. Cataloluk, O.; Gogebakan, B. Presence of drug resistance in intestinal lactobacilli of dairy and human origin in Turkey. *FEMS Microbiol. Lett.* **2004**, *236*, 7–12. [CrossRef]
47. Gad, G.F.; Abdel-Hamid, A.M.; Farag, Z.S. Antibiotic resistance in lactic acid bacteria isolated from some pharmaceutical and dairy products. *Braz. J. Microbiol.* **2014**, *45*, 25–33. [CrossRef]
48. Drago, L.; Mattina, R.; Nicola, L.; Rodighiero, V.; De Vecchi, E. Macrolide resistance and in vitro selection of resistance to antibiotics in Lactobacillus isolates. *J. Microbiol.* **2011**, *49*, 651. [CrossRef] [PubMed]

Publisher's Note: MDPI stays neutral with regard to jurisdictional claims in published maps and institutional affiliations.

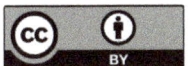

© 2020 by the authors. Licensee MDPI, Basel, Switzerland. This article is an open access article distributed under the terms and conditions of the Creative Commons Attribution (CC BY) license (http://creativecommons.org/licenses/by/4.0/).

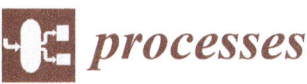

Article

Enterococcal Species Associated with Slovak Raw Goat Milk, Their Safety and Susceptibility to Lantibiotics and Durancin ED26E/7

Andrea Lauková *, Valentína Focková and Monika Pogány Simonová

Institute of Animal Physiology, Centre of Biosciences of the Slovak Academy of Sciences, Šoltésovej 4-6, 040 01 Košice, Slovakia; fockova@saske.sk (V.F.); simonova@saske.sk (M.P.S.)
* Correspondence: laukova@saske.sk; Tel.: +421-557-922-964

Citation: Lauková, A.; Focková, V.; Pogány Simonová, M. Enterococcal Species Associated with Slovak Raw Goat Milk, Their Safety and Susceptibility to Lantibiotics and Durancin ED26E/7. *Processes* **2021**, *9*, 681. https://doi.org/10.3390/pr9040681

Academic Editor: Nevijo Zdolec

Received: 24 March 2021
Accepted: 10 April 2021
Published: 13 April 2021

Publisher's Note: MDPI stays neutral with regard to jurisdictional claims in published maps and institutional affiliations.

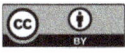

Copyright: © 2021 by the authors. Licensee MDPI, Basel, Switzerland. This article is an open access article distributed under the terms and conditions of the Creative Commons Attribution (CC BY) license (https://creativecommons.org/licenses/by/4.0/).

Abstract: Goat milk has become a popular item of human consumption due to its originality. Enterococci are ubiquitous bacteria, and they can also be found in traditional dairy products. This study focuses on the safety of enterococci from Slovak raw goat milk and on their susceptibility to lantibiotic bacteriocins and durancin ED26E/7, which has not previously been studied. Biofilm formation ability in enterococci, virulence factor genes, enzyme production and antibiotic profile were investigated. Samples of raw goat milk (53) were collected from 283 goats in Slovakia. MALDI-TOF mass spectrometry identified three enterococcal species: *Enterococcus faecium*, *E. hirae* and *E. mundtii*, with dominant occurrence of the species *E. faecium*. Low-grade biofilm formation ability ($0.1 \leq A_{570} < 1.0$) was found in four strains of *E. faecium*. *Gelatinase*, *hyaluronidase*, *aggregation substance* and *enterococcal surface protein* genes were absent in these enterococci. Gene *efaAfm* (adhesin) was detected in five *E. faecium* strains. However, it was not detected in biofilm-forming strains. Enterococci detected in Slovak raw goat milk were found not to have pathogenic potential; four strains even produced high amounts of useful β-galactosidase. The strains were susceptible to lantibiotic bacteriocin treatment and to durancin ED26E/7 as well, which represents original information in dairy production.

Keywords: raw goat milk; enterococcal species; safety; virulence factor; bacteriocins

1. Introduction

Enterococci are widespread microorganisms which can also be found in many traditional dairy products [1,2]. They belong in a community of lactic acid-producing bacteria which forms part of a controversial group of dairy bacteria [3], because antibiotic-resistant enterococci or virulence-factor genes possessing enterococci can cause human health disorders [4]. In general, based on the previous studies, the prevalent enterococcal species in raw milk have been found to be *Enterococcus faecium*, *E. faecalis* and *E. durans* [3]. Knowledge of these properties is required in order to reduce the pathogenic enterococcal strains from dairy production, and to eliminate the transfer of virulence-factor genes to other strains. It is also essential to find possible ways of eliminating them; the application of bacteriocins represents a promising approach, especially those with a broad antimicrobial spectrum [5–7]. The beneficial use of bacteriocins for these purposes has been confirmed several times under in vitro, in situ and in vivo studies [8,9]. As previously mentioned, the controversial character of enterococci lies in their beneficial as well as undesirable properties, especially in the beneficial production of proteinaceous antimicrobial substances—namely, enterocins [5]. In the past, the inhibition of *Staphylococcus aureus* SA1 in skim milk and yoghurt production was confirmed using enterocin CCM 4231 and its anti-listerial potential [8]. Moreover, enterocins showed benefit in food-producing animals. In broiler rabbits, they stimulated phagocytic activity, and increased the reparation ability of enterocytes [9]. An increase in body weight [10] was also noted, as was the reduction of *Eimeria* oocysts [9]. The most frequently studied enterocins are those produced by representatives of the species

E. faecium [5,11,12], but bacteriocins produced by strains of E. durans [13,14] have also been reported. Enterocins are known to have an inhibition spectrum against more or less related bacteria [15].

Gallidermin is a polypeptide containing the amino acid residues lanthionine, β-methyllanthionine or α,β-didehydroamino acids, which are able to build intramolecular thioether bridges. This antimicrobial bacteriocin was first found in the strain *Staphylococcus gallinarum* TU 3928. Members of this group of bacteriocins are called lantibiotics [16], to which nisin also belongs, and is commercially available. Nisin has garnered significant influence in the food industry since its discovery as an alternative biopreservative [17]. Nisin and gallidermin act predominantly against Gram-positive bacteria [16].

Milk has become a regular component of human consumption due to its originality. In Slovakia, in addition to raw cow milk and products made from it, ewe milk and its products are also very popular among consumers [18]. The consumption of raw goat milk and goat milk products has also increased because of their benefit to humans [19]. The specificity of goat milk lies, for example, in the fact that it has more abundant immunoglobulin content than human milk. Goat milk is also higher in calcium content compared with cow milk, contains trace elements and is full of vitamins. The content of some fatty acids in goat milk is also high [20].

Regarding the potential involved, this study focuses on the safety aspects of enterococci isolated from raw goat milk, with the intention of testing properties such as biofilm formation ability, virulence-factor genes, enzyme production, antibiotic profile, as well as hemolysis and/or deoxyribonuclease activity. To investigate the in vitro possibility of eliminating enterococci with pathogenic character, their susceptibility to the commercial lantibiotic bacteriocins nisin and gallidermin was tested, as well as their susceptibility to durancin ED26E/7 (identified in our laboratory), produced by the *Enterococcus durans* ED26E/7 strain from ewe milk lump cheese [14].

2. Materials and Methods

2.1. Sampling, Strains Isolation and Identification

Raw goat milk (a total of 53 samples) was collected from healthy goats in central and eastern regions of Slovakia. Altogether 283 goats were sampled. Samples (51) were taken from individual goats, and two pooled milk samples were taken from 132 goats. Treatment of the milk samples followed the standard microbiological method specified by the International Organization for Standardization (ISO 6887-1:2017). First, they were diluted in Ringer solution (1:9, Merck, Germany). Then dilutions were plated onto M-Enterococcus medium (Difco, Lawrence, KS, USA). Agar plates were cultivated at 37 °C for 48 h. Different pure colonies were picked up and submitted for identification. Matrix-assisted laser desorption ionization time-of-flight mass spectrometry (MALDI-TOF MS, Brucker Daltonics, Billerica, MD, USA) was applied to identify isolates. This identification method is based on bacterial protein "fingerprints" [21]. The preparation of bacterial cell lysates followed the producer's instructions, and results evaluation was based on the MALDI Biotyper 3.0 identification database (Bruker Daltonics). Allocation of isolates was performed according to their MALDI-TOF MS score evaluation based on highly probable species identification (score 2.300–3.000), secure genus identification/probable species identification (2.000–2.299) and probable genus identification (1.700–1.999). Reference strains included in the Bruker Daltonics database were used as positive controls. Strains evaluated with the same score value (identical) were excluded. Enterococci were inoculated on M-Enterococcus medium (Difco, USA), and were stored using the Microbank system (Pro-Lab Diagnostic, Richmond, BC, Canada).

2.2. Biofilm Formation

The ability of the identified strains to form biofilms was checked using Congo red agar [22]. Agar plates were inoculated with the tested enterococci, incubated at 37 °C overnight and checked at 48 and 72 h. Biofilm formation was assessed through the presence of black colonies with dry crystalline consistency. Negative strains remained pink. The positive, standard biofilm-forming control strain was *Streptococcus equi* subsp. *zooepidemicus* CCM 7316 (kindly provided by Dr. Eva Styková, University of Veterinary Medicine and Pharmacy in Košice, Slovakia). Growth of the strains tested was compared with the growth of the positive control strain.

Moreover, the biofilm-forming ability of enterococci was assayed using the quantitative plate method according to Chaieb et al. [23] and Slížová et al. [24]. One colony of each strain picked up from Brain heart medium after cultivation for 24 h at 37 °C (Difco, NJ, USA) was inoculated into 5 mL Ringer solution (pH 7.0, 0.75% w/v). The suspension obtained corresponded to 1×10^8 cfu/mL. A 100 µL volume from that dilution was transferred into 10 mL of Brain heart infusion (BHI, Difco, USA). A 200 µL volume of dilution was transferred into microtiter plate wells (Greiner ELISA 12 Well Strips, 350 µL, flat bottom, Frickenhausen GmbH, Germany). The plate was incubated for 24 h at 37 °C, and the biofilm formed in the microtiter plate wells was washed twice with 200 µL of deionized water. It was then dried at 25 °C for 40 min. The attached bacteria were stained for 30 min at 25 °C with 200 µL of 0.1% (w/v) crystal violet in deionized water, and the dye solution was aspirated away. The wells in the microtiter plate were washed twice with 200 µL of deionized water. After water removal, the plate was dried for 30 min at laboratory temperature. The dye bound to the adherent biofilm was extracted with 200 µL of 95% ethanol. A 150 µL volume was transferred from each well into a new microplate well to measure absorbance in nm (A_{570}). An Apollo 11 Absorbance Microplate reader LB 913 (Apollo, Berthold Technologies, Oak Ridge, TN, USA) was used for this measurement. Testing was repeated in two independent runs with 12 replicates. Sterile BHI was used in each testing, serving as negative control. Biofilm-forming strain *Streptococcus equi* subsp. *zooepidemicus* CCM 7316 (kindly provided by Dr. Eva Styková, University of Veterinary Medicine and Pharmacy in Košice, Slovakia) served as positive control. Biofilm formation was evaluated as highly positive ($A_{570} \geq 1.0$), low-grade positive ($0.1 \leq A_{570} < 1.0$) or negative ($A_{570} < 0.1$), as per Chaieb et al. [23] and Slížová et al. [24].

2.3. Virulence-Factor Gene Detection

Genes for five virulence factors were tested. PCR amplification with the primers and conditions used followed the protocols according to Kubašová et al. [25] and Lauková et al. [26]. The genes tested were as follows: *gelE* (gelatinase), *esp* (enterococcal surface protein), *efaAfm* (*E. faecium* adhesin), *hylEfm* (hyaluronidase) and *agg* (aggregation substance). The PCR products were separated by means of agarose gel electrophoresis (1.2% w/v, Sigma-Aldrich, Saint Louis, USA) with 1 µL/mL content of ethidium bromide (Sigma-Aldrich) using 0.5× TAE buffer (Merck, Darmstadt, Germany). PCR fragments were visualized with UV light. The strains *E. faecalis* 9Tr1 (our strain, Lauková et al. [27]) and *E. faecium* P36 (Dr. Semedo-Lemsaddek, University in Lisbon, Portugal) were positive controls. The PCRs were carried out in 25 µL volume. Testing mixture consisted of 1× reaction buffer, 0.2 mmol/L of deoxynucleoside triphosphate, 3 mmol MgCl$_2$, 1 µmol/L of each primer, 1 U of Taq DNA polymerase, and 1.5 µL of DNA template. The cycling conditions followed the protocol as previously reported by Kubašová et al. [25] and Lauková et al. [26].

2.4. Enzyme Activity and Antibiotic Resistance Tests

Enzyme activity in the identified enterococci was tested with the API-ZYM system (BioMérioux, Marcy l'Etoile, France). Enzymes involved in the kit were as follows: alkaline phosphatase, esterase (C4), esterase lipase (C8), lipase (C14), leucine arylamidase, valine arylamidase, cystine arylamidase, trypsin, α-chymotrypsin, acid phosphatase, naphtol-AS-BI-phosphohydrolase, α-galactosidase, β-galactosidase, β-glucuronidase, α-glucosidase, β-glucosidase, N-acetyl-β-glucosaminidase, α-mannosidase and α-fucosidase. An amount of 65 µL McFarland standard one inoculum was transferred into each well of the test plate. Incubation was performed for 4 h at 37 °C. After that time, the reagents Zym A and Zym B were added and enzyme activity was evaluated. Color intensity values from 0 to 5 and their relevant values in nanomoles (nmoL) were assigned for each reaction according to the color chart supplied with the kit.

Following the EFSA rules for analyzing antibiograms, the CLSI [28] method was used together with antibiotic disks. Twelve antibiotics in disks (Oxoid, USA) were tested according to the suppliers' recommendation: clindamycin (Da 2 µg); novobiocin (Nov, 5 µg); ampicillin (Amp, 10 µg); erythromycin, azithromycin (Ery, Azm, 15 µg); streptomycin (S, 30 µg); chloramphenicol, rifampicin, vancomycin, tetracycline, kanamycin (C, R, Van, Tc, Kan, 30 µg) and gentamicin (Gn, 120 µg). Overnight culture (100 µL) of broth culture medium (BHI) was spread on Blooded BH agar (Difco, USA). Disks were placed on the agar surface. Then, plates were cultivated at 37 °C for 24 h. Inhibition zones were evaluated and expressed in millimeters according to the disk suppliers' recommendations.

2.5. Hemolysis and Deoxyribonuclease Activity

Hemolysis formation was checked by inoculating the cultures onto BH agar (Difco, USA) supplemented with 5% defibrinated sheep blood. Plates were incubated at 37 °C for 24 h. The presence/absence of clear zones around the bacterial colonies was read as α- and β-hemolysis, and negative strains featured γ-hemolysis [29].

To determine deoxyribonuclease activity, each strain was spread onto the surface of DNase agar (Oxoid, USA), and the agar plates were incubated for 24 h at 37 °C. The production of deoxyribonuclease can be evaluated on this medium. Colonies producing DNase hydrolyze the deoxyribonucleic acid (DNA) within the medium. After flooding and acidifying the agar with 1 N HCl, the DNA precipitated out; the agar became turbid with clear zones around the DNase-positive colonies.

2.6. Susceptibility of Enterococci to Nisin, Gallidermin and Durancin ED26E/7

Nisin was supplied in the product Nisaplin (Aplin and Barret, United Kingdom), in which activity of nisin is 1,000,000 IU. The dosage of nisin used in testing was prepared according to Lauková et al. [10]. Gallidermin, the pure substance supplied by Enzo Life Sci. Corporation USA, (MW2069.4), was used at a concentration of 0.5 mg/mL in 2 µL doses. This was decided based on the results of previous studies. Raw durancin ED26E/7 was prepared according to the previous report by Lauková et al. [14]. Enterococci were tested using the agar diffusion method [30]. Brain heart infusion supplemented with 1.5% agar (BHIA, Difco, Lawrence, KN, USA) was used for the bottom layer. For the overlay, 0.7% BHIA enriched with 200 µL of the indicator culture strain was used (A_{600} up to 1.0). Bacteriocin dilution (10 µL of nisin and durancin, 2 µL of gallidermin) in phosphate buffer (pH 6.5, ratio 1:1) was dropped on the surface of soft agar with each tested enterococcal strain, and the plates were incubated at 37 °C for 18 h. Clear inhibition zones around the doses of diluted bacteriocins were read. Inhibition activity was expressed in arbitrary units per milliliter (AU/mL), as the reciprocal of the highest two-fold dilution of bacteriocins demonstrating complete growth inhibition of the tested strain. Tests were performed twice. Positive control was the principal indicator, fecal *Enterococcus avium* EA5 strain (from piglet, isolated in our laboratory); inhibition activity reached up to 102,400 AU/mL.

3. Results

3.1. Strains Identification, Biofilm Formation and Virulence-Factor Detection

Among 53 samples of raw goat milk from two regions of Slovakia, three enterococcal species were detected: *E. faecium*, *E. hirae* and *E. mundtii*. The species *E. faecium* dominated with 11 strains (Table 1), followed by one strain of *E. hirae* and one strain of *E. mundtii*. Five out of eleven *E. faecium* strain species were evaluated, with highly probable species identification (2.300–3.000), five *E. faecium* strains as well as one strain of *E. hirae* were identified with evaluation corresponding to secure genus identification/probable species identification (2.000–2.299). *E. faecium* EF16/1 and *E. mundtii* EM 2/2 were identified with scores corresponding to probable genus identification (1.700–1.999).

Table 1. Enterococci detected in raw goat milk, with biofilm formation and virulence factor gene detection.

Strain	Score	Congo/72	Biofilm	*efaAfm* Gene
EF3/2	2.315	ng	0.081 (0.02)	nt
EF4/1	2.310	ng	0.090 (0.02)	nt
EF6/2	2.201	ng	0.092 (0.03)	+
EF10/2	2.006	ng	0.076 (0.07)	+
EF11/1	2.317	ng	0.089 (0.03)	ng
EF12/1	2.225	+	0.119 (0.35)	ng
EF14/2	2.257	+	0.108 (0.32)	ng
EF15/1	2.345	ng	0.089 (0.03)	+
EF16/1	1.894	+	0.113 (0.34)	+
EF18/1	2.352	ng	0.087 (0.03)	nt
EF23	2.200	+	0.101 (0.32)	ng
EH21	2.197	ng	0.90 (0.04)	+
EM2/2	1.939	ng	0.075 (0.01)	nt

EF: *Enterococcus faecium*; EH: *E. hirae*; EM: *E. mundtii*; ng: negative; nt: not tested; +: positive; Biofilm: absorbance at 570 nm (SD); Score: MALDI-TOF mass spectrometry evaluation score.

Using Congo red agar, most enterococci did not form biofilm (Table 1); however, four strains of *E. faecium* were found to have biofilm formation ability (EF12/1, EF14/2, EF16/1 and EF23). The strains *E. hirae* EH21 and *E. mundtii* EM2/2 were negative. The strains with biofilm formation ability not detected on Congo red agar were not biofilm-forming, as tested with the quantitative method (A_{570} < 0.1). Four biofilm-forming *E. faecium* strains were evaluated with low-grade positive biofilm formation ability (Table 1; $0.1 \leq A_{570} < 1.0$).

Enterococci were *gelE* gene, *hylEfm* gene, *esp* gene and *agg* gene absent. Gene *efaAfm* (*E. faecium* adhesin) was present in five *E. faecium* strains (EF6/2, EF10/2, EF15/1, EF16/1 and *E. hirae* EH21, Table 1), however this gene was not detected in biofilm-forming strains.

3.2. Enzyme Production, Antibiotic Susceptibility, Hemolysis and Deoxyribonuclease Activity

E. faecium strains EF3/2, EF4/1, EF6/2, EF11/1, EF16/1 and EF23 did not produce enzymes when tested. The strains EF 10/2, EF12/1 and EF14/2 showed high volumes of the enzyme β-galactosidase (30 nmoL, 20 nmoL), and in strains EF15/1 and EH21 we measured 40 nmoL of β-galactosidase. EH21 also showed 30 nmoL for β-glucosidase, and 20 nmoL was found in the case of strain EF15/1. The strains EF14/2, EF12/1 and EF10/2 produced β-glucosidase only at the 5 nmoL level. The other enzymes were not produced at all, or only in slight amounts (5–10 nmoL). Trypsin, α-chymotrypsin and naphtol-AS-BI-phosphohydrolase were not produced.

Enterococci from raw goat milk were mostly susceptible to antibiotics including ampicillin (inhibition zone size in range 11–18 mm), penicillin (14–20 mm), erythromycin (12–20 mm), vancomycin (15–20 mm), gentamicin (12–20 mm), chloramphenicol (12–25 mm), tetracycline (20–30 mm) and rifampicin (11–22 mm, except EF11/1 and EM2/2). However, they were resistant to kanamycin and clindamycin (Da). Most strains were also resistant to streptomycin (except EF18/1 and EM2/2). *E. faecium* EF6/2, EF14/2 and EF15/1 were resistant to Da and streptomycin (S 30 µg). EF10/2 was monoresistant (S 30 µg) as was EF16/1 (Azm, Table 2). *E. faecium* EF11/1 was resistant to four antibiotics (Da, Nv, S and R). The strains EF12/1 and EF18/1 were resistant to three antibiotics: Da, Nv (novobiocin 5 µg) and to S or Azm (EF18/1, Table 2). *E. mundtii* EM2/2 was found to have resistance against Da, S and R. *E. hirae* EH21 was susceptible to antibiotics; however, it possessed the *efaAfm* gene. EF16/1 was Azm resistant, biofilm-forming and possessed the *efaAfm* gene. Enterococci were hemolysis negative (γ-hemolysis) and deoxyribonuclease negative.

Table 2. Antibiotic profile of enterococci detected in raw goat milk.

Strains	6/2	10/2	11/1	12/1	4/2	15/1	16/1	18/1	EH21	EM2/2
Da (2 µg)	R	20 S	R	R	R	R	25 S	R	25 S	R
Nv (5 µg)	15 S	15 S	R	R	17 S	11 S	16 S	15 S	16 S	15 S
Azm (15 µg)	13 S	16 S	12 S	14 S	13 S	12 S	R	R	12 S	11 S
S (30 µg)	R	R	R	R	R	R	14 S	R	14 S	R

Da: clindamycin; Nv: novobiocin; Azm: azithromycin; S: streptomycin; S: susceptible, size of inhibition zone (mm); R: resistant, no inhibition zone. All strains were resistant to kanamycin. Strains were susceptible to vancomycin (15–20 mm), tetracycline (20–30 mm), chloramphenicol, rifampicin (30 µg), gentamicin (120 µg; 12–20 mm), erythromycin (15 µg), penicillin (10 IU; 14–20 mm), and ampicillin (10 µg; 11–18 mm).

3.3. Susceptibility of Enterococci to Treatment with Nisin, Gallidermin and Durancin ED26E/7

Enterococci were susceptible to treatment with bacteriocins. Pure-form nisin and gallidermin inhibited the growth of enterococci with high inhibition activity. Using nisin, inhibition activity ranged from 6400 AU/mL (against EF16/1) to 204,800 AU/mL (Table 3). Enterococci growth was inhibited using gallidermin, with activity from 200 to 204,800 AU/mL. Although durancin ED26E/7 was used only in raw substance, enterococci growth was still inhibited, but lower inhibition activity was measured (100–25,600 AU/mL, Table 3).

Table 3. Susceptibility of enterococci from raw goat milk to bacteriocins (AU/mL).

Strains	Nis	Gal	ED26E/7
EF6/2	204,800	204,800	25,600
EF10/2	51,200	204,800	6400
EF11/1	204,800	204,800	400
EF12/1	204,800	204,800	800
EF14/2	51,200	204,800	6400
EF15/1	12,800	3200	100
EF16/1	6400	6400	25,600
EF18/1	51,200	51,200	25,600
EF23	102,400	102,400	25,600
EH21	12,800	200	100

EF: *Enterococcus faecium*; EH: *E. hirae*. *E. mundtii* EM2/2, EF3/2 and EF4/2 were not tested. Nis: nisin; Gal: gallidermin; ED26E/7: durancin; AU/mL: arbitrary units per milliliter.

The biofilm-forming strain EF16/1 (Azm resistant, possessing the *efaAfm* gene) was inhibited with bacteriocins at a lower activity (AU/mL) than other strains (Table 3). Though still susceptible to all antibiotics used, *E. hirae* EH21, was the least susceptible to bacteriocins.

4. Discussion

In general, milk is an important nutritional component for populations worldwide, but it is also a useful matrix for a variety of bacteria [31]. Enterococci occur naturally in dairy products, as previously reported [19,32], with *E. faecium* and *E. faecalis* being predominant. Shirru et al. [33] also found a high prevalence of *E. faecium* strains in raw goat milk in Sardinia. Teržič-Vidojević et al. [3] reported that the most prevalent enterococcal species in milk and cheeses were *E. faecium*, *E. faecalis* and *E. durans*. Usually, enterococci detected in milk are from the same or related cluster/group, which is reflected in the results of our study. Enterococcal species detected in the present study are from the same bacterial cluster/group (i.e., *E. faecium*, following gene similarity 16S rRNA analysis) [34]. Regarding raw goat milk or raw milk in general, enterococci can come from animal handling [35]. MALDI-TOF MS spectrometry has emerged as a tool for rapid microbial identification. This analytical technique is based on the ionization of chemical compounds into charged molecules, and the ratio of their mass to charge is measured [36]. Although it has been shown that enterococci have little value as hygiene indicators in the industrial processing of foods, it is necessary to evaluate them in terms of their safety [34].

Hyaluronidase and gelatinase are hydrolytic enzymes which are involved in virulence factor levels in enterococci. Gelatinase gelE is an extracellular zinc metallo-endopeptidase. This gene is mostly secreted by *E. faecalis* [37]. The *gelE* gene is located on the chromosome. It is regulated in a cell-density-dependent manner, and hydrolyses gelatin, casein, hemoglobin and another bioactive peptides. Hyaluronidase is a degradative enzyme associated with tissue damage which acts on hyaluronic acid [38], and is encoded by the chromosomal *hyl* gene. The enterococci we tested were *gelE* and *hyl* gene absent. The presence of the *agg* gene (aggregation substance) increases the hydrophobicity of the enterococcal cell surface. It is a pheromone-inducible surface glycoprotein which mediates aggregate formation during conjugation [37]. This gene was also absent in enterococci isolated from raw goat milk. In this study, the *efaAfm* gene (*E. faecium* adhesin gene for adhesion to collagen) was detected in five strains of *E. faecium*. While it has not yet been conclusively shown to contribute to pathogenesis in animal experiments, it may nevertheless pose a safety risk [39].

Latassa et al. [38] reported that some Esp-negative *E. faecalis* strains were able to produce biofilms after receiving plasmid transfer of the *esp* gene. The enterococci we tested were *esp* gene absent, and only four strains were able to form biofilm (low-grade biofilm-forming ability). Mannu et al. [40] reported that the *esp* gene was absent in dairy isolates, which could be explained by the fact that Esp factor is thought to promote adhesion, colonization and evasion of the immune system. It is also thought to play some role in antibiotic resistance [6]. Enterococci can be intrinsically resistant towards antibiotics such as cephalosporins, β-lactams, sulfonamides and low levels of clindamycin and aminoglycosides [41]. As a result of their intrinsic resistance, antibiotic-resistant strains can frequently be found. Although phenotype testing for antibiotic resistance/susceptibility was performed in this study, enterococci from Slovak raw goat milk were mostly susceptible to antibiotics, except clindamycin (2 μg), kanamycin and streptomycin (30 μg).

Biofilm formation can also contribute to enterococcal pathogenicity and can act as persistent sources of contamination, leading to hygiene problems in food products [42]. However, in our tests, only low-grade ability to form biofilm was detected in four enterococcal strains. In addition, enterococci were hemolysis-negative (γ-hemolysis) and were DNase negative as well.

In our results from enterococci testing, it is particularly promising that the strains involved appear not to be pathogenic (mostly free of virulence-factor gene occurrence), and some of them even produce high amounts of β-galactosidase. This enzyme is used in the dairy industry for the production of lactose-free milk intended for lactose-intolerant humans [43]. Moreover, no production or only slight amounts (5 nmoL) of undesirable enzymes (e.g., naphtol-AS-BI-phosphohydrolase) were measured in our testing.

Although enterococci detected in Slovak raw goat milk appear not to be pathogenic, their potential elimination using bacteriocins is indicated. The strains were susceptible to bacteriocin treatment. The inhibition of enterococci through treatment with enterocins was also reported in our previous studies, for example, against fecal enterococci possessing virulence-factor genes [44]. Enterocin was also reported to inhibit *L. monocytogenes* and *S. aureus* in milk products [8], and the inhibitory effect of nisin in broiler rabbits was demonstrated after its application in drinking water [10].

5. Conclusions

The representatives of three enterococcal species in Slovak raw goat milk were found not to have pathogenic potential. The originality of this study, however, is in the fact that enterococci were susceptible to lantibiotic bacteriocin treatment, and to durancin ED26E/7 as well. Some of enterococci even produce high amounts of the β-galactosidase enzyme, which is used in the dairy industry for the production of lactose-free milk intended for lactose-intolerant people.

Author Contributions: Conceptualization, A.L.; methodology, M.P.S. and A.L.; investigation, V.F., M.P.S. and A.L.; resources, A.L.; data curation, A.L.; writing—original draft preparation, A.L.; project administration, A.L.; funding acquisition, A.L. All authors have read and agreed to the published version of the manuscript.

Funding: This research was funded by the Slovak Research and Development Agency under contract no. APVV-17-0028.

Data Availability Statement: All data included in this study are available upon request by contacting the corresponding author.

Acknowledgments: We are grateful to Dana Melišová for her skillful laboratory work. We also thank Martin Tomáška and MiroslavOlošta for providing goat milk samples. Our cordial thanks also go to Andrew Billingham for English language proofing. Some information regarding strains is involved in preparing the "Safety and Control of Foods" conference, Piešťany, June 2021. Some results regarding the strain EM 2/2 were presented in *IJERPH*, **2020**, *17*, 9504; doi:10.3390/ijerph17249504 by Lauková et al.

Conflicts of Interest: The authors declare no conflict of interest.

References

1. Gelsomino, R.; Vancanneyt, M.; Condon, S.; Swings, J.; Cogan, T.M. Enterococcal diversity in the environment of an Irish cheddar–type cheesemaking factory. *Int. J. Food Microbiol.* **2001**, *17*, 177–188. [CrossRef]
2. Lauková, A.; Focková, V.; Pogány Simonová, M. *Enterococcus mundtii* isolated from Slovak raw goat milk and its bacteriocinogenic potential. *Int. J. Environ. Res. Public Health* **2020**, *17*, 9504. [CrossRef] [PubMed]
3. Terzič-Vidojevič, A.; Veljovič, K.; Begovič, J.; Filipič, B.; Popovič, D.; Tolinački, M.; Miljkovič, M.; Kojič, M.; Golič, N. Diversity and antibiotic susceptibility of authchtonnous dairy enterococci isolates:are they safe candidates for authochtonnous starter cultures? *Front. Microbiol.* **2015**, *6*, 954. [CrossRef] [PubMed]
4. Valenzuela, A.J.S.; Benomar El Bakoli, N.; Abriouel, H.; Rosario, L.L.; Veljovic, K.; Martinez-Tanamero, M.; Topisarovic, L.; Gálvez, A. Virulence factors, antibiotic resistance and bacteriocins in enterococci from asrtisan foods of animal origin. *Food Control* **2009**, *20*, 381–385. [CrossRef]
5. Franz, C.M.A.P.; Van Belkum, M.J.; Holzapfel, W.H.; Abriouel, H.; Gálvez, A. Diversity of enterococcal bacteriocins and their grouping in a new classification scheme. *FEMS Microbiol. Rev.* **2007**, *31*, 293–310. [CrossRef]
6. Foulquié-Moreno, M.R.; Sarantinopoulos, P.; Tsakalidou, E.; De Vuyst, L. The role and application of enterococci in food and health. *Int. J. Food Microbiol.* **2006**, *106*, 1–24. [CrossRef]
7. Lauková, A.; Pogány Simonová, M.; Focková, V.;Ološta, M.; Tomáška, M.; Dvorožňáková, E. Susceptibility to bacteriocins in biofilm-forming, variable staphylococci isolated from local ewe's milk lump cheeses. *Foods* **2020**, *9*, 1335. [CrossRef]
8. Lauková, A.; Czikková, S.; Dobránsky, T.; Burdová, O. Inhibition of *Listeria monocytogenes* and *Staphylococcus aureus* by enterocin CCM 4231 in milk products. *Food Microbiol.* **1999**, *16*, 93–99. [CrossRef]
9. Pogány Simonová, M.; Chrastinová, Ľ.; Lauková, A. Autochtonnous strain *Enterococcus faecium* EF2019 (CCM7420), its bacteriocin and their beneficial effects in broiler rabbits—A review. *Animals* **2020**, *10*, 1188. [CrossRef] [PubMed]
10. Lauková, A.; Chrastinová, Ľ.; Plachá, I.; Kandričáková, A.; Szabóová, R.; Strompfová, V.; Chrenková, M.; Čobanová, K.; Žitňan, R. Beneficial effect of lantibiotic nisin in rabbit husbandry. *Probiotics Antimicrob. Proteins* **2014**, *6*, 41–46. [CrossRef]
11. Lauková, A.; Mareková, M.; Javorský, P. Detection and antimicrobial spectrum of a bacteriocin-like substance produced by *Enterococcus faecium* CCM4231. *Lett. Appl. Microbiol.* **1993**, *16*, 257–260. [CrossRef]
12. Mareková, M.; Lauková, A.; Skaugen, M.; Nes, I.F. Isolation and characterization of a new bacteriocin termed enterocin M, produced by environmental isolate *Enterococcus faecium* AL41. *J. Ind. Microbiol. Biotechnol.* **2007**, *34*, 533–537. [CrossRef] [PubMed]
13. Du, L.; Liu, F.; Zhao, P.; Zhao, T.; Doyle, M.P. Characterization of *Enterococcus durans* 152 bacteriocins and their inhibition of *Listeria monocytogenes* in ham. *Food Microbiol.* **2017**, *68*, 97–103. [CrossRef] [PubMed]
14. Lauková, A.; Chrastinová, Ľ.; Kandričáková, A.; Ščerbová, J.; Plachá, I.; Pogány Simonová, M.; Čobanová, K.; Formelová, Z.; Ondruška, Ľ.; Strompfová, V. Bacteriocin substance durancin-like ED26E/7 and its experimental use in broiler rabbits. *Maso* **2015**, *5*, 56–59. (In Slovak)
15. Nes, I.F.; Diep, D.B.; Moss, M.O. Enterococcal bacteriocins and antimicrobial proteins that contribute to niche control. In *Enterococci from Commensals to Leading of Drug Resistant Infection*; Massachussets Eye and Ear: Boston, MA, USA, 2014; pp. 1–34.
16. Bierbaum, G.; Goetz, F.; Peschel, A.; Kupke, T.; van de Kamp, M.; Sahl, H.G. The biosynthesis of the lantibiotics epidermin, gallidermin, pep 5 and epilancin K7. *Antonie van Leeuwenhoek* **1996**, *69*, 119–127. [CrossRef]
17. Shin, J.M.; Won Gwak, J.; Pachiappan, K.; Fenno, C.H.J.; Rickard, A.H.; Kapila, Y.L. Biomedical applications of nisin. *J. Appl. Microbiol.* **2016**, *120*, 1449–1465. [CrossRef]
18. Herian, M. Benefit of sheep milk products to human health. *Milk Lett. (Mlékařské Listy)* **2014**, *143*, 1–6. (In Slovak)
19. Lauková, A.; Kandričáková, A.; Bino, E.; Tomáška, M.;Ološta, M.; Kmeť, V.; Strompfová, V. Some safety aspects of enterococci isolated from Slovak lactic acid dairy product "žinčica". *Folia Microbiol.* **2020**, *65*, 79–85. [CrossRef]

20. Uhrín, V.; Lauková, A.; Jančová, A.; Plintovič, V. *Mlieko a Mliečna Žľaza (in Slovak) Milk and Mammary Gland*; Publ. No. 92; Faculty of Natural Sciences of the University Constantinus Philosophus: Nitra, Slovakia, 2002; pp. 5–167. ISBN 80-8050-511-X.
21. Alatoom, A.A.; Cunningham, S.A.; Ihde, S.; Mandrekar, J.; Patel, R. Comparison of direct colony method versus extraction method for identification of Gram-positive cocci by use of Bruker Biotyper matrix-assissted laser desorption ionization-time of flight mass spectrometry. *J. Clin. Microbiol.* **2011**, *49*, 2868–2873. [CrossRef]
22. Freeman, D.J.; Falkiner, F.R.; Keane, C.T. New method for detecting slime production by coagulase-negative staphylococci. *J. Clin. Pathol.* **1989**, *42*, 872–874. [CrossRef]
23. Chaieb, K.; Chehab, O.; Zmantar, T.; Rouabhia, M.; Mahdouani, K.; Bakhrouf, A. In vitro effect of pH and ethanol on biofilm formation by clinical *ica*-positive *Staphylococcus epidermidis* strains. *Ann. Microbiol.* **2007**, *57*, 431–437. [CrossRef]
24. Slížová, M.; Nemcová, R.; Maďar, M.; Hádryová, J.; Gancarčíková, S.; Popper, M.; Pistl, J. Analysis of biofilm formation by intestinal lactobacilli. *Can. J. Microbiol.* **2015**, *61*, 437–466. [CrossRef]
25. Kubašová, I.; Diep, D.B.; Ovčinnikov, K.V.; Lauková, A.; Strompfová, V. Bacteriocin production and distribution of bacteriocin-encoding genes in enterococci from dogs. *Int. J. Antimicrob. Agents* **2020**, *55*, 105859. [CrossRef]
26. Lauková, A.; Stromfpvá, V.; Ščerbová, V.; Pogány Simonová, M. Virulence factor genes incidence among enterococci from sewage sludge in eastern Slovak following safety aspect. *BioMed Res. Int.* **2019**, 2735895. [CrossRef]
27. Lauková, A.; Strompfová, V.; Kandričáková, A.; Ščerbová, J.; Semedo-Lemsaddek, T.; Miltko, R.; Belzecki, G. Virulence factors genes in enterococci isolated from beavers (*Castor fiber*). *Folia Microbiol.* **2015**, *60*, 151–154. [CrossRef]
28. CLSI. *Clinical Laboratory Standard Institute Guideline 2020/2020 Performance Standards for Antimicrobial Susceptibility Testing M100S*, 30th ed.; CLSI: Wayne, PA, USA, 2020.
29. Semedo-Lemsaddek, T.; Santos, M.A.; Lopes, M.F.S.; Figueiredo Marques, J.J.; Barreto Crespo, M.T.; Tenreiro, R. Virulence factors in food, clinical and reference Enterococci: A common trait in the genus? *Syst. Appl. Microbiol.* **2003**, *26*, 13–22. [CrossRef]
30. De Vuyst, L.; Callewaert, R.; Pot, B. Characterization of antagonistic activity of *Lactobacillus amylovorus* DCE471 and large-scale isolation of its bacteriocin amylovorin L471. *Syst. Appl. Microbiol.* **1996**, *19*, 9–20. [CrossRef]
31. Ur Rahman, U.; Shahzad, T.; Sahar, A.; Ishaq, A.; Khan, M.; Zahoor, T.; Aslam, S. Recapitulating the competence of novel and rapid monitoring tools for microbial documentation in food systems. *LWT Food Sci. Technol.* **2016**, *67*, 62–66. [CrossRef]
32. Giraffa, G. Functionality of enterococci in dairy producvts. *Int. J. Food Microbiol.* **2003**, *88*, 215–222. [CrossRef]
33. Schirru, S.; Todorov, S.D.; Favaro, L.; Mangia, N.P.; Basaglia, M.; Casella, S.; Comunian, R.; Gombossy de Melo Franco, D. Sardinian goat's milk as a source of bacteriocinogennic potential protective cultures. *Food Control* **2020**, *25*, 309–320. [CrossRef]
34. Franz, C.M.A.P.; Huch, M.; Abriouel, H.; Holzapfel, W.; Gálvez, A. Enterococci as probiotics and their implications in food safety. *Int. J. Food Microbiol.* **2011**, *151*, 125–140. [CrossRef]
35. Bhardwaj, A.; Malik, R.K.; Chauhan, P. Functional and safety aspects of enterococci in dairy foods. *Ind. J. Microbiol.* **2008**, *48*, 317–325. [CrossRef]
36. Singhal, N.; Kumar, M.; Kanaujia, P.K.; Virdi, J.S. Maldi-Tof mass spectrometry, an emerging technology for microbial identification and diagnosis. *Front. Microbiol.* **2015**, *6*, 791. [CrossRef]
37. Koch, S.; Hufnagel, M.; Theilacker, C.; Huebner, J. Enterococcal infections: Host response, therapeutic, and prophylactic possibilities. *Vaccine* **2004**, *22*, 822–830. [CrossRef]
38. Latassa, C.; Solano, C.; Penadés, J.R.; Lasa, I. Biofilm associated proteins. *Comptes Rendus Biol.* **2006**, *329*, 849. [CrossRef]
39. Fisher, K.; Phillips, C. The ecology, epidemiology and virulence of *Enterococcus*. *Microbiology* **2009**, *155*, 1749–1757. [CrossRef]
40. Mannu, L.; Paba, A.; Daga, E.; Comunian, R.; Zanetti, S.; Dupré, I.; Sechi, L.A. Comparison of the incidence of virulence determinants and antibiotic resistance between *Enterococcus faecium* strains of dairy, animal and clinical origin. *Int. J. Food Microbiol.* **2003**, *88*, 291–304. [CrossRef]
41. Jett, B.D.; Huycke, M.M.; Gilmore, M.S. Virulence in enterococci. *Clin. Microbiol.* **1994**, *7*, 462–478. [CrossRef]
42. Giaouris, E.; Heir, E.; Hebraud, M.; Chorianopoulos, N.; Langsrud, S.; Moretro, T.; Habimana, O.; Desvaux, M.; Renier, S.; Nychas, G.J. Attachment and biofilm formation by foodborne bacteria in meat processing encvironments: Causes, implications, role of bacterial interactions and control by alternative novel methods. *Meat Sci.* **2014**, *97*, 298–309. [CrossRef]
43. Zeinat, K.; Nawal Magdy, M.; Farahat, M.G. Optimization of culture conditions for production of β-galactosidase by *Bacillus megaterium* NM56 isolated from raw milk. *Res. J. Pharm. Biol. Chem. Sci.* **2016**, *7*, 366–376.
44. Lauková, A.; Kandričáková, A.; Ščerbová, J.; Strompfová, V. Enterococci isolated from farm ostriches and their relation to enterocins. *Folia Microbiol.* **2016**, *61*, 275–281. [CrossRef] [PubMed]

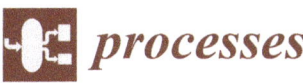

Article

Biogenic Amine Content in Retailed Cheese Varieties Produced with Commercial Bacterial or Mold Cultures

Nevijo Zdolec [1], Tanja Bogdanović [2], Krešimir Severin [3], Vesna Dobranić [1], Snježana Kazazić [4], Jozo Grbavac [5], Jelka Pleadin [6], Sandra Petričević [2] and Marta Kiš [1,*]

[1] Department of Hygiene, Technology and Food Safety, Faculty of Veterinary Medicine, University of Zagreb, 10 000 Zagreb, Croatia; nzdolec@vef.hr (N.Z.); vdobranic@vef.hr (V.D.)
[2] Veterinary Center Split, Croatian Veterinary Institute, 21 000 Split, Croatia; t.bogdanovic.vzs@veinst.hr (T.B.); petricevic.vzs@veinst.hr (S.P.)
[3] Department of Forensic and State Veterinary Medicine, Faculty of Veterinary Medicine, University of Zagreb, 10 000 Zagreb, Croatia; severin@vef.hr
[4] Division of Physical Chemistry, Ruđer Bošković Institute, 10 000 Zagreb, Croatia; Snjezana.Kazazic@irb.hr
[5] Faculty of Agriculture and Food Technology, University of Mostar, 88 000 Mostar, Bosnia and Herzegovina; grbavac.jozo@gmail.com
[6] Laboratory for Analytical Chemistry, Croatian Veterinary Institute, 10 000 Zagreb, Croatia; pleadin@veinst.hr
* Correspondence: mkis@vef.hr; Tel.: +385-1-2390-199

Abstract: Biogenic amines (BAs) are considered a potential microbiological toxicological hazard in aged cheese. Risk mitigation strategies include good hygiene practice measures, thermal treatment of milk and the use of competitive dairy cultures. The aim of this study was to evaluate the amount of BAs—tryptamine, β-phenylethylamine, putrescine, cadaverine, histamine, tyramine, spermidine and spermine—in the core and rind of cheeses ripened by bacteria ($n = 61$) and by mold cultures ($n = 8$). The microbial communities were counted, and the dominant lactic acid bacteria (LAB) were identified, corresponding to the BA concentrations. The total BA content was highest in the core of semi-hard cheeses (353.98 mg/kg), followed by mold cheeses (248.99 mg/kg) and lowest in hard cheeses (157.38 mg/kg). The highest amount of BAs was present in the rind of cheeses with mold (240.52 mg/kg), followed by semi-hard (174.99 mg/kg) and hard cheeses (107.21 mg/kg). Tyramine was the most abundant BA, represented by 75.4% in mold cheeses, 41.3% in hard cheese and 35% of total BAs in semi-hard cheeses. Histamine was present above the defined European maximum level (ML) of 100 mg/kg in only two semi-hard and three hard cheeses. High amount of BAs (above 600 mg/kg) in cheeses, mainly tyramine, were associated with the presence of *Enterococcus durans*, while negligible BA concentrations were found in cheeses ripened with *Lacticaseibacillus rhamnosus*, *Lactococcus lactis* or *Lacticaseibacillus paracasei* cultures. This study has shown that retailed cheese varieties produced with commercial bacterial or mold cultures have acceptable levels of biogenic amines with respect to consumers.

Keywords: biogenic amines; enterococci; lactobacilli; lactococci; ripened cheese

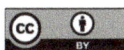

1. Introduction

Biogenic amines (BAs) are low molecular weight compounds associated with the decarboxylation activity of microorganisms in fermented foods, particularly in aged cheeses [1,2]. Although they have a number of different regulatory functions in animal and plant tissues, as well as in microbial cells, their formation and sustainability in food requires attention, as consumption of foods containing large amounts of BAs may have serious toxicological consequences [2]. They are formed during the ripening and storage of cheese, and the factors affecting BA formation are pH, salt concentration, bacterial activity, humidity, storage temperature and ripening time [3]. In ripened cheeses, the BAs detected in the highest concentrations are tyramine, cadaverine, histamine and putrescine [2,4]. The total numbers of BAs in different cheeses available in the market vary considerably, reaching values up to 257.71 mg/kg for hard cheese and 384.33 mg/kg for semi-hard cheese in Korea [5], 407.8 mg/kg in hard and semi-hard cheeses and up to 327.5 mg/kg in mold-ripened cheese in Croatia [6] and 1875.43 mg/kg in hard cheese in Egypt [7]. However, BA concentrations can further increase during cheese storage, i.e., during shelf life. In a recent study, Dabadé et al. [8] reported a tyramine concentration of 1029 mg/kg in a semi-hard cheese at its expiry date. Hard cheeses were found to have stable and high concentrations of tyramine and histamine (1025 mg/kg) during storage, while most of the amines were found to be tyramine and cadaverine (1306 mg/kg) in blue cheeses. The average concentrations of BAs in the samples of hard cheeses (e.g., Parmesan) were found to be significantly higher than in other cheeses.

Some of these high amounts have toxicological significance for consumers when compared with the set European maximum level (MLs) of histamine in fish of 100 mg/kg [9]. Indeed, for other foods, especially fermented foods, there are no regulated set MLs for individual or total amines. Kandasamy et al. [5] reported that although the tolerance limit for toxic amines in cheese is 200 mg/kg, amine amounts of 1889.75 mg/kg and 1237.80 mg/kg were found in extra hard cheeses (imported Pecorino Romano and Grana Padano). Ladero et al. [10] consider the difficulty in establishing MLs for individual amines in foods, given insufficient toxicological studies; since different BAs are simultaneously present in foods, the MLs of 750–900 mg/kg can be recommended. On the other hand, Ladero et al. [10] emphasize that it would be reasonable to set preventive "m"/"M" limits of 200 and 500 mg of individual BA per kg for foods that are likely to contain many BAs, such as cheese.

Given the aminogenic potential of microorganisms, it is crucial to know the composition of the cheese microbiota and the possible relationship between microbial activity and the formation of amines in them. The microbiological properties of cheese depend on the type of cheese, i.e., hygiene and production technology, especially heat treatment of milk and the use of dairy cultures [4,11]. The microbiota of raw milk under poor hygiene conditions may contain pathogenic bacteria, such as *Listeria monocytogenes* and *Staphylococcus aureus*, but also fecal or environmental contaminating bacteria, such as coliforms or enterococci [12–14]. In this context, coliform bacteria and lactic acid bacteria (LAB), mainly enterococci, are responsible for the formation of biogenic amines in unprocessed dairy products [15,16]. In general, higher microbiological contamination, i.e., a higher total number of bacteria in raw material, may also cause a higher formation of BAs in cheese made from unpasteurized milk [7].

However, correlations between microbiological counts and end-of-storage concentrations of BAs (or trends in BA concentrations) have generally been weak for various commercially available foods, including cheese [8]. This can be explained by the low sensitivity of culturable microbiological methods and the reduction of microbial populations during extended cheese storage. For example, Vrdoljak et al. [17] reported a reduction of LAB in hard cheeses from 7 logs to 2 logs during 450 days of storage as well as from 6.2 to 4.6 logs in semi-hard cheeses during a 270-day period. In addition to the total number of microorganisms, such as aerobic mesophiles, psychrotrophs, enterobacteria or LAB, involved in the production of BAs, the presence of certain species may be important in evaluating the accumulation or even reduction of BAs in cheese. The microbial species most commonly associated with the formation of the major BAs found in food are *Enterococcus faecalis, E. faecium* and *E. durans* (tyramine), while others, such as *Lactiplantibacillus plantarum, Latilactobacillus sakei, Lactiplantibacillus pentosus* and *Pediococcus acidilactici*, degrade tyramine and histamine [18,19].

One of the strategies to reduce the formation of BAs in ripening cheeses is to make use of competitive dairy cultures due to their possible inhibitory effect on amine-producing bacteria.

Therefore, the objective of this study was to select retail semi-hard and hard cheeses produced with the addition of bacterial cultures to gain insight into the amounts of BAs and their possible connection with microbial populations. The study assumed that cheeses incorporated with bacterial dairy cultures would contain low amounts or at least toxicologically acceptable amounts of the main BAs. In addition, the quantities of BAs in commercially available soft cheeses aged with selected mold cultures were evaluated.

2. Materials and Methods

2.1. Cheese Samples

Samples of local and imported cheeses ($n = 69$) in the original retail packaging were collected for the study (Table 1). All cheeses were made from pasteurized cow, goat or sheep milk and ripened by mold or bacterial cultures. The mold-ripened cheese group consisted of surface-ripened white mold cheeses (Brie/Camembert type, $n = 3$) and internal mold-ripened, blue-veined cheeses (Gorgonzola type, $n = 5$). The group of semi-hard cheeses ($n = 18$) consisted of internal-bacterial ripened varieties (Trappist, Dutch type) from 6 producers. The group of hard cheeses ($n = 43$) consisted of the cheese type Parmigiano-Reggiano, internal-bacterial ripened cheeses with or without additional ingredients (fruits and wine), and came from 9 producers.

Table 1. Characteristics of retail cheese selected in this study.

Cheese Group, Number of Samples	Properties (Microbial Cultures Involved in Ripening)	Milk
Mold-ripened ($n = 8$)	Surface-ripened—white mold cheese—Brie/Camembert type (Germany, $n = 3$)	Cow
	Internal mold—blue-veined—Gorgonzola type (Croatia, Italy, Netherlands, $n = 5$)	Cow ($n = 4$) Goat ($n = 1$)
Semi-hard cheese ($n = 18$)	Internal-bacterial ripened—Trappist type (Croatia, * $n = 5$, ** $n = 1$; Bosnia and Herzegovina, *** $n = 5$); Internal-bacterial ripened, rennet (Bosnia and Herzegovina, **** $n = 5$) Dutch type cheese (New Zealand, ***** $n = 2$)	Cow
Hard cheese ($n = 43$)	Parmigiano-Reggiano cheese type (Croatia, * $n = 5$), Internal-bacterial ripened (Bosnia and Herzegovina, ** $n = 5$, Croatia, *** $n = 10$), Internal-bacterial ripened (Croatia, **** $n = 15$)	Cow
		Cow ($n = 5$), goat ($n = 5$), ewe ($n = 5$)
	Internal-bacterial ripened (Croatia, ***** $n = 3$)	Ewe
	(Croatia, ****** $n = 1$)	Ewe
	(Croatia, ******* $n = 1$),	Cow
	Internal-bacterial ripened with wine (Croatia, ******** $n = 1$),	Cow
	Internal-bacterial ripened with apricot/cranberry (Great Britain, ********* $n = 2$)	Cow

* Different asterisks represent different producers within cheese group.

2.2. Microbiological Analyses

For microbiological analysis, 25 g of cheese was taken after sterile separation of the surface layers of the product. The test sample was diluted in 225 mL of buffered peptone water (Biolife, Milano, Italy) and homogenized at 200 rpm for 2 min (Stomacher, Seward, UK). Serial decimal dilutions were then prepared to determine the number of aerobic mesophilic bacteria, LAB, enterococci, yeasts and molds, enterobacteria and *Escherichia coli*. The number of aerobic mesophilic bacteria was determined on plate count agar (PCA, bioMerieux, Craponne, France) by incubation at 30 °C for 72 h. The number of LAB was determined on de Man–Ragosa–Sharpe agar (MRS, Merck, Darmstadt, Germany) and incubated at 30 °C for 24–48 h, and enterococci on Compass Enterococcus agar chromogenic medium (BIOKAR, Beauvais, France) by incubation at 37 °C for 24 h. The number of yeasts and molds was determined on oxytetracycline glucose yeast agar (Merck, Darmstadt, Germany) by incubation at 25 °C for 48–72 h. The number of *E. coli* was determined on rapid *E. coli* chromogenic medium (BIOKAR, Beauvais, France) and incubated at 37 °C for 24 h, and enterobacteria on violet red bile agar with glucose (VRBG, Merck, Darmstadt, Germany) by incubation at 37 °C for 24 h. Before counting, catalase, oxidase and coagulase tests were performed for LAB, enterobacteria and staphylococci, respectively. The results are expressed as logarithmic values of the numbers of colonies per gram of cheese ($\log_{10}$ CFU/g).

2.3. Identification of Dominant Lactic Acid Bacteria (LAB)

Colonies grown on MRS agar were selected from the highest sample dilutions of semi-hard and hard cheeses and determined to the species level by matrix-assisted laser desorption/ionization time-of-flight mass spectrometry (MALDI-TOF MS, Bruker Daltonik, Bremen, Germany). A sample for MALDI TOF MS analysis was prepared following the extended direct transfer procedure recommended by the manufacturer (Bruker Daltonik, Bremen, Germany). A single colony was smeared onto a 96-spot polished steel target plate, applied with 1 µL of 70% formic acid (Fisher Scientific, Madrid, Spain) and dried at room temperature. Each sample was overlaid with 1 µL of MALDI matrix (a saturated solution of α-cyano-4-hydroxycinnamic acid, HCCA, Bruker Daltonik, Bremen, Germany) in 50% acetonitrile and 2.5% trifluoroacetic acid (Sigma-Aldrich, St. Louis, MO, USA) and air dried at room temperature. Mass spectra were automatically generated using a microflex LT MALDI TOF mass spectrometer (Bruker Daltonik, Bremen, Germany) operated in the linear positive mode within a mass range of 2000–20,000 Da. The instrument was calibrated using a Bruker bacterial test standard. Recorded mass spectra were processed with the MALDI Biotyper 3.0 software package (Bruker Daltonik, Bremen, Germany), using standard settings. The MALDI Biotyper output is a log score value in the range 0–3.0, representing the probability of correct identification of the isolate, computed by comparison of the peak list for an unknown isolate with the reference spectrum in the database. The identification criteria used were as follows: a score of 2300–3000 indicated highly probable species level identification, a score of 2000–2299 indicated secure genus identification with probable species identification, a score of 1700–1999 indicated probable identification to the genus level and a score of <1700 was considered unreliable.

2.4. Determination of Biogenic Amines (BA)

The 8 biogenic amines studied (cadaverine—CAD, histamine—HIS, phenylethylamine PHE, putrescine—PUT, spermidine—SPD, spermine—SPM, tryptamine—TRP and tyramine—TYR) were detected and quantified by high performance liquid chromatography, using a diode array detector (G1315B DAD, Agilent Technologies, Santa Clara, CA, USA) at 254 nm, with 550 nm as a reference after precolumn derivatization with dansyl chloride, as described by Eerola et al. [20] and Bogdanović et al. [6]. The extraction of a 5 g homogenized cheese sample (from both the cheese core and cheese rind) was performed in 50 mL 0.4 mol/L perchloric acid. A total of 250 µL of an internal standard solution (1,7 heptanediamine, 1000 mg/L) was added to the homogenized sample prior to the extraction with 0.4 M perchloric acid. One mililiter of perchloric cheese extract was derivatized according to Bogdanović et al. [6]. Each food sample was analyzed in triplicate, the BA content stated herein represents the mean of these three parallel analyses. BA concentrations are expressed as mg/kg (wet weight).

Chromatographic separation of 8 BAs of interest was performed by high-performance liquid chromatography in combination with a diode array detector (HPLC-DAD, Agilent Technologies 1200 Series HPLC, Santa Clara, CA, USA), according to Bogdanović et al. [6]. The precise instrument module details and HPLC-DAD parameters were as described in Supplementary Materials. The compounds were quantified using internal calibration curves plotted for each BA and covering 8 concentration levels ranging from 0.25–500 mg/kg. The method used for biogenic amine determination in cheese was validated according to the criteria laid down in the EC Regulation No. 333/2007. The performance assessment criteria included the applicability, limit of detection (LOD), limit of quantification (LOQ), precision (RSDr), specificity, linearity and recovery. The precision of the method was assessed at three concentration levels under repeatable conditions (RSDr). Cheese samples were spiked at the concentrations of 50, 100 and 250 mg/kg in triplicate. The presence or absence of matrix effects was identified using calibration curves and a fixed amount of internal 1,7 heptane diamine (HEP) standard (50 mg/kg) obtained with matrix-matched calibration standards and calibration solutions in the solvent. Internal quality control was pursued with each analytical batch using the available quality control material (canned fish T27137QC, HIS assigned value: 212 ± 30 mg/kg, Fapas, York, England), and was carried out by virtue of spiking the cheese samples so as to obtain the concentration of 100 mg/kg. Within each analytical series, the reference materials and the spiked cheese samples were analyzed in duplicate and checked for recovery. The applied analytical method fulfils all methodological requirements set out under the EC Regulation No. 333/2007 and can therefore be considered as suitable for the determination of 8 BAs in food groups under this study. The results concerning linearity, LOD, LOQ, recovery and RSDr are presented in Supplementary Materials.

2.5. Statistical Analysis

Statistical analysis of the results was performed using standard descriptive statistical methods (Statistica 13.5, TIBCO Software, Palo Alto, Santa Clara, CA, USA) by determining the arithmetic mean (x) with the standard deviation (SD) and the minimum (min) and maximum (max) values. Kruskal–Wallis analysis of variance at the 0.05 probability level was used to determine statistically significant differences between the cheeses, and post-hoc analysis was used to determine the differences between each group as well as between different producers within the same cheese group. The correlation between the individual values of BAs and bacteria was determined with the Spearman correlation coefficient (r_s).

3. Results and Discussion

Results of microbiological analyses of soft cheeses with mold, semi-hard and hard cheeses are presented in Table 2.

Table 2. Microbial population counts ($\log_{10}$ CFU/g) in different cheese types.

Microorganisms	Mold-Ripened (n = 8)		Semi-Hard Cheese (n = 18)		Hard Cheese (n = 43)	
	Mean ± SD	Min/Max	Mean ± SD	Min/Max	Mean ± SD	Min/Max
Aerobic mesophilic bacteria	5.74 ± 1.42 [a]	4.04–7.77	7.30 ± 0.46 [ab]	6.25–7.95	5.74 ± 1.80 [b]	2.00–7.80
Enterococci	4.18 ± 1.21	2.69–5.90	5.03 ± 2.20	2.00–8.55	5.20 ± 1.14	2.30–6.60
Lactic acid bacteria	6.84 ± 1.09	5.00–7.90	7.57 ± 0.97 [a]	4.00–8.50	6.60 ± 0.93 [a]	4.69–8.00
Yeasts and molds	6.49 ± 1.30 [ab]	5.00–7.69	3.43 ± 1.48 [a]	2.00–7.95	3.10 ± 1.07 [b]	2.00–6.00
Enterobacteriaceae	2.38 ± 0.49	1.69–3.00	3.06 ± 0.56	2.00–3.50	2.23 ± 0.91	1.00–3.80
Staphylococci	3.73 ± 0.65	2.69–4.47	3.82 ± 0.98	2.69–6.30	3.80 ± 0.34	2.84–4.38
Escherichia coli	<2.00	<2.00	<2.00	<2.00	3.81 ± 0.23	3.50–4.07

Values in the same row marked with the same letter denote statistically significant differences ($p < 0.05$).

Table 2 shows that LABs are the dominant microbiota in all investigated cheese types, with an average number of 6–7 $\log_{10}$ CFU/g. A stable population of enterococci (members of the LAB group) in the number of 4–5 $\log_{10}$ CFU/g and an equal number of coagulase-negative staphylococci (3.5 $\log_{10}$ CFU/g) is also observed. The number of yeasts and molds is almost the same in semi-hard and hard cheeses, and significantly different ($p < 0.05$) from their number in soft cheeses (6.49 $\log_{10}$ CFU/g) due to the technological process involving molds. *Enterobacteriaceae* were found occasionally in all cheese groups, but the result was mainly related to individual producers. Surprisingly, *E. coli* was also present in hard cheeses (n = 5) from one producer. A wide range of results can be observed in all studied microbial populations grouped by cheese types (soft cheese with mold, semi-hard cheese, and hard cheese), indicating significant differences in production technology, dairy culture activity or hygienic production conditions. Microbiological changes in/on cheese during production or storage depend on various factors, such as production technology and type of cheese (pasteurization of milk or raw milk, use of dairy cultures, acidity and ripening), physicochemical properties of cheese and storage conditions [21]. Lactic acid bacteria are technologically the most important microorganisms in cheese production, and their numbers in the studied cheeses depends on the type of product, i.e., conditioned application of dairy cultures. Further development of LABs in cheese during storage depends on the type of cheese, consequently it generally decreases in semi-hard and hard cheeses and increases in soft cheeses [17]. As far as contaminating microorganisms are concerned, the findings of enterobacteria, *E. coli* and enterococci may indicate poor quality of the raw material used and deficiencies in the milk pasteurization. Bacterial thermoresistance is well documented, especially in enterococci, thus lower temperatures applied in cheese technology may not affect their population, as was the case for the amine-producing *Enterococcus durans* in the study by Ladero et al. [22]. Moreover, the possibility of the contamination of the cheese after processing should not be ignored. Enterococci are known to be controversial ubiquitous bacteria, and their presence in cheese is not necessarily an indicator of fecal contamination [23]. In any case, these microorganisms have a high aminogenic potential and can influence the content of biogenic amines, especially tyramine in cheese [24]. Coagulase-negative staphylococci were found in equal numbers in all cheese types and, together with LAB, are technologically/safety important dairy bacteria, but health risks can be expected if resistant and amine- or enterotoxin-producing strains are present [25,26].

Table 3 shows the determined concentration of each BA analyzed in the core and rind of soft cheeses with mold, semi-hard cheeses and hard cheeses. The total content of amines in the core was highest in semi-hard cheese (353.98 mg/kg), followed by mold cheese (248.99 mg/kg) and lowest in hard cheese (157.38 mg/kg). Among the surface samples, the highest content of BA was present in cheese with mold (240.52 mg/kg), followed by semi-hard (174.99 mg/kg) and hard cheese (107.21 mg/kg). In contrast to soft and hard cheeses, in the semi-hard cheese group, the amounts of all amines were higher in the middle than in the rind, and statistically significant differences were found for putrescine, tyramine and spermine ($p < 0.05$). Considering the amounts of BAs in the core and rind of the cheese, a positive correlation was found in all three cheese groups: soft cheese ($r = 0.97$), semi-hard cheese ($r = 0.78$) and hard cheese ($r = 0.91$). It is well known that BA content varies between different aged cheeses, within the same cheese type and within cheese parts [27]. This study shows that BA content is lowest in hard, long-ripened cheeses, which contrasts with other findings claiming a direct effect of ripening time and intense proteolytic changes with accumulation of BAs [7,27,28]. The obtained differences between mentioned studies may be explained by the competitiveness of lactic starters against aminogenic non-starter lactic acid bacteria (NSLAB). For example, the lowest BA content represented only by cadaverine (<0.61–1.28 mg/kg) and spermidine (<0.39–2.57 mg/kg) was found in a Croatian variety of Parmigiano-Reggiano cheese aged for 1–3 years, and the dominant isolated culture was *Lacticaseibacillus rhamnosus*, without enterococci. Shalabi et al. [29]. demonstrated high anti-tyramine potential of *Lacticaseibacillus rhamnosus* against tyrosine decarboxylase gene carrying strains isolated from cheese. In general, the total content of BA in cheese ripened by bacteria or molds in this study is 2–5 times lower than the toxicological limits proposed by Ladero et al. [10].

Table 3. Biogenic amine content in retailed cheese varieties ripened with mold or bacterial dairy cultures.

BAs	Mold-Ripened ($n = 8$)				Semi-Hard Cheese ($n = 18$)				Hard Cheese ($n = 43$)			
	Core		Rind		Core		Rind		Core		Rind	
	Mean	Min–Max	Mean	Min–Max	Mean	Min–Max	Mean	Min–Max	Mean	Min–Max	Mean	Min–Max
TRP	<0.77	<0.77	<0.77	<0.77	<0.77	<0.77	<0.77	<0.77	9.01 [a]	1.56–23.89	5.58 [a]	2.55–19.62
β-PHE	42.90	1.43–84.38	30.03	<0.63–84.18	46.55	1.07–130.59	18.81	1.39–55.25	16.05	0.64–52.44	24.55	10.08–92.85
PUT	6.38	0.64–30.53	4.39	1.01–8.04	15.93 [Aa]	1.37–95.21	9.78 [Ba]	0.80–62.56	3.31 [A]	<0.59–11.63	2.28 [B]	<0.59–9.13
CAD	2.57 [A]	<0.61–5.38	3.70 [B]	2.35–4.70	64.22 [A]	0.76–436.68	38.17 [B]	<0.61–292.80	19.48 [A]	<0.61–119.38	12.77	<0.61–83.85
HIS	7.05	0.74–13.99	6.23	2.59–13.07	87.82	13.5–248.55	40.83	4.17–127.01	28.35	<0.59–116.42	20.96	<0.59–85.90
TYR	183.97	0.97–710.5	185.13	1.86–62.75	129.96 [Aa]	2.30–767.03	55.13 [a]	<0.89–376.66	72.60 [A]	1.33–236.33	36.69	<0.89–142.81
SPD	6.12	1.75–16.58	11.04	1.62–22.24	7.03 [A]	3.35–17.90	11.65	0.50–66.53	5.35 [A]	<0.39–21.70	4.38	<0.39–18.17
SPM	<1.01	<1.01	7.32	<1.01–15.64	2.47 [a]	<1.01–9.02	<1.01 [a]	<1.01–1.15	3.23	<1.01–5.12	10.05	<1.01–10.96

n—number of samples, BAs—biogenic amines, TRP—tryptamine, β-PHE—β-phenylethylamine, PUT—putrescine, CAD—cadaverine, HIS—histamine, TYR—tyramine, SPD—spermidine, SPM—spermine. Values expressed as < (less than) denoted values lower than the method detection limit. Uppercase letters (A or B) in the same row denote statistically significant differences ($p < 0.05$) between cheese groups (mold-ripened, semi-hard, hard cheese); a lowercase letter (a) in the same row denotes statistically significant differences ($p < 0.05$) between core and rind within the cheese group.

Regarding the percentage of each BA in total BAs, tyramine was the most abundant amine, accounting for 75.4% in mold cheese, 41.3% in hard cheeses, and 35% of the total amines in semi-hard cheeses. These results are consistent with other studies showing that tyramine is the dominant BA in various cheeses, including those investigated in this study [6,29]. The average tyramine content was below 200 mg/kg; however, there were large differences between individual samples and even within the same cheese varieties, as previously reported [6]. Among individual samples, a mold-ripened cheese and a semi-hard cheese had the highest tyramine concentrations of 762.75 mg/kg and 767.03 mg/kg, respectively.

The other BAs were present across a wide spectrum in all the cheeses studied, except for tryptamine, which was found in low concentrations only in hard cheeses. The second most abundant amine in semi-hard and hard cheeses was histamine, and its content was higher in the core than in the rind in both cheeses, which was found by Marijan et al. [1] in hard cheeses, but without statistical significance in case of this study ($p > 0.05$). Although no statistically significant differences were found in histamine content between cheeses, significant differences were observed within the group of semi-hard cheeses between the producers of these cheeses ($p < 0.05$). Only two semi-hard cheeses and three hard cheeses had histamine amounts above the 100 mg/kg; defined in the European Union as ML level [30]. Histamine is the most toxicologically significant of all amines and frequently exceeds maximum food safety levels, and its concentrations are reported to be higher in raw milk cheeses than in processed cheeses [27]. The greatest differences between cheese types were found for cadaverine, whose amounts were 2.57–64.22 mg/kg in the core of the cheese and 3.70–38.17 mg/kg in the rind ($p < 0.05$). The high variability of cadaverine concentrations in cheese was also reported by Bunka et al. [31]; however, maximum values determined in this study were several times lower.

Comparing the association of the BAs found with the isolated microbiota, numerous differences were found according to the cheese group and within the producer. In the semi-hard cheese group, the number of enterococci and staphylococci was found to be statistically significantly positively correlated ($r > 0.6$) with the amount of ß-phenylethylamine, histamine and tyramine, but differed between producers. LAB as well as yeasts and molds reduce the synthesis of certain BAs, which has been confirmed by a negative correlation factor (r > −0.49) in the case of histamine, putrescine and tyramine. The amine-reducing ability of LABs, such as lactobacilli or lactococci, has been previously reported in aged cheese [32,33]. In this study, *Lacticaseibacillus paracasei* and *Lactococcus lactis* were isolated from LAB populations (highest dilutions) of semi-hard and hard cheeses, which had a very low total amount of BAs. It can be assumed that their dominance in the cheese microbiota resulted in lower BA content in the cheeses from this study.

In the group of semi-hard cheeses, the number of *Enterobacteriaceae* correlated positively with the value of putrescine (r = 0.81) and negatively affected spermin synthesis (r = −0.76). In hard cheeses, their number correlated with the value of ß-phenylethylamine, histamine and spermine. The aminogenic potential of enterobacteria is well known, especially in the formation of putrescine, and their presence is the consequence of poor hygienic practices in cheese production [10]. Although enterococci are associated with a risk of biogenic amines, their differential effect on BA synthesis has been observed. For example, at a concentration of 4.5 $\log_{10}$ CFU/g, their number was significantly positively correlated with the amount of spermidine (r = 0.9) in semi-hard cheeses from the same producer, while a negative correlation was observed in another cheese at a concentration of 8 $\log_{10}$ CFU/g (r = −0.94). Such discrepancies may be due to different production conditions, as inappropriate environmental factors, such as pH, temperature or salt concentration, may influence BA production [34]. The most common species of enterococci in milk are *Enterococcus faecium*, *Enterococcus durans* and *Enterococcus faecalis*, most of which have been identified as tyramine and putrescine producers [10,35]. In this study, in two varieties of semi-hard and hard cheeses, the dominant species within LAB was *E. durans*, and these cheeses had the highest BA values, of which tyramine was found at the highest concentrations. Considering that enterococci are usually not present in the function of starter cultures and that their introduction is the result of subsequent contamination (NS-LAB), it is expected that this is the case with analysis of these types of cheeses, which confirm the presence of high numbers of enterobacteria and staphylococci in them.

4. Conclusions

This study has shown that retailed cheese varieties produced with commercial bacterial or mold cultures have acceptable levels of biogenic amines with respect to consumers. The microbial communities examined were generally associated with the accumulation or reduction of BAs in the cheese samples, firstly, by the dominance of enterococci and, secondly, by the dominance of lactobacilli or lactococci. This was evident in individual producers of semi-hard cheeses, where the largest populations of enterococci and staphylococci correlated with the highest concentrations of BAs, especially tyramine, histamine, cadaverine, putrescine and β-phenyletilamine. Unlike enterococci, the presence of LAB is likely to be associated with a reduction in the synthesis of BAs, but, given the many variations in their counts, to confirm this it will be necessary to evaluate their activity patterns in the controlled production of different cheeses. According to the obtained results, the aminogenic or amine-reducing capacity of the bacterial strains collected from the cheeses in this study will be further investigated.

Supplementary Materials: The following supporting information can be downloaded at: https://www.mdpi.com/article/10.3390/pr10010010/s1, Reagents and materials for biogenic amines determination and quantification; HPLC-DAD analysis; Table S1: Selected performance indicators of the method in use: linearity, limit of detection (LOD), limit of quantification (LOQ), recovery and precision (RSD_r).

Author Contributions: Conceptualization, N.Z. and V.D.; methodology, T.B. and N.Z.; software, K.S. and M.K.; validation, T.B. and S.P.; formal analysis, N.Z., T.B., S.K. and S.P.; investigation, M.K., K.S. and N.Z.; resources, J.G. and V.D.; data curation, K.S. and M.K.; writing—original draft preparation, N.Z.; writing—review and editing, J.P., T.B. and M.K.; project administration, N.Z. and M.K. All authors have read and agreed to the published version of the manuscript.

Funding: This research was funded by by the EU Operational Program Competitiveness and Cohesion 2014–2020 project "Potential of microencapsulation in cheese production" K.K.01.1.1.04.0058 and European Regional Development Fund, project "CEKOM 3LJ" K.K.01.2.2.03.0017.

Institutional Review Board Statement: Not applicable.

Informed Consent Statement: Not applicable.

Data Availability Statement: Not applicable.

Conflicts of Interest: The authors declare no conflict of interest.

References

1. Marijan, A.; Džaja, P.; Bogdanović, T.; Škoko, I.; Cvetnić, Ž.; Dobranić, V.; Zdolec, N.; Šatrović, E.; Severin, K. Influence of ripening time on the amount of certain biogenic amines in rind and core of cow milk Livno cheese. *Mljekarstvo* **2014**, *64*, 59–69.
2. Sahu, L.; Panda, S.K.; Paramithiotis, S.; Zdolec, N.; Ray, R. Biogenic Amines in Fermented Foods: Overview. In *Fermented Foods Part I. Biochemistry and Biotechnology*; Montet, D., Ray, R., Eds.; CRC Press Taylor & Francis Group: Boca Raton, FL, USA, 2016; pp. 318–332.
3. Ruiz-Capillas, C.; Herrero, A.M. Impact of biogenic amines on food quality and safety. *Foods* **2019**, *8*, 62. [CrossRef]
4. Benkerroum, N. Biogenic amines in dairy products: Origin, incidence, and control means. *Compr. Rev. Food Sci. Food Saf.* **2016**, *15*, 801–826. [CrossRef]
5. Kandasamy, S.; Yoo, J.; Yun, J.; Kang, H.B.; Seol, K.-H.; Ham, J.-S. Quantitative analysis of biogenic amines in different cheese varieties obtained from the Korean domestic and retail markets. *Metabolites* **2021**, *11*, 31. [CrossRef]
6. Bogdanović, T.; Petričević, S.; Brkljača, M.; Listeš, I.; Pleadin, J. Biogenic amines in selected foods of animal origin obtained from the Croatian retail market. *Food Addit. Contam. Part A* **2020**, *37*, 815–830. [CrossRef]
7. Ma, J.-K.; Raslan, A.A.; Elbadry, S.; El-Ghareeb, W.R.; Mulla, Z.S.; Bin-Jumah, M.; Abdel-Daim, M.M.; Darwish, W.S. Levels of biogenic amines in cheese: Correlation to microbial status, dietary intakes, and their health risk assessment. *Environ. Sci. Pollut. Res. Int.* **2020**, *27*, 44452–44459. [CrossRef]
8. Dabadé, S.D.; Jacxsens, L.; Miclotte, L.; Abatih, E.; Devlieghere, F.; De Meulenaer, B. Survey of multiple biogenic amines and correlation to microbiological quality and free amino acids in foods. *Food Control* **2021**, *120*, 107497. [CrossRef]
9. European Commission. Commission Regulation (EC) No 2073/2005 of 15 November 2005 on microbiological criteria for foodstuffs. *Off. J. Eur. Union.* **2005**, *338*, 1–26.
10. Ladero, V.; Calles-Enríquez, M.; Fernández, M.; Alvarez, M.A. Toxicological effects of dietary biogenic amines. *Curr. Nutr. Food Sci.* **2010**, *6*, 145–156. [CrossRef]
11. Doeun, D.; Davaatseren, M.; Chung, M.S. Biogenic amines in foods. *Food Sci. Biotechnol.* **2017**, *26*, 1463–1474. [CrossRef]
12. Zdolec, N.; Jankuloski, D.; Kiš, M.; Hengl, B.; Mikulec, N. Detection and Pulsed-Field Gel Electrophoresis Typing of Listeria monocytogenes Isolates from Milk Vending Machines in Croatia. *Beverages* **2019**, *5*, 46. [CrossRef]
13. Mikulec, N.; Špoljarić, J.; Zamberlin, Š.; Krga, M.; Radeljević, B.; Plavljanić, D.; Horvat Kesić, I.; Zdolec, N.; Dobranić, V.; Antunac, N. The investigation of suitability of raw milk consumption from vending machines in Croatia. *J. Cent. Eur. Agric.* **2019**, *20*, 1076–1088. [CrossRef]
14. Kiš, M.; Kolačko, I.; Zdolec, N. Unprocessed milk as a source of multidrug-resistant *Staphylococcus aureus* strains. *Acta Vet. Brno* **2021**, *90*, 357–363. [CrossRef]
15. Burdychova, R.; Komprda, T. Biogenic amine-forming microbial communities in cheese. *FEMS Microbiol. Lett.* **2007**, *276*, 149–155. [CrossRef]
16. Ladero, V.; Fernández, M.; Calles-Enríquez, M.; Sánchez-Llana, E.; Cañedo, E.; Martín, M.C.; Alvarez, M.A. Is the production of the biogenic amines tyramine and putrescine a species-level trait in enterococci? *Food Microbiol.* **2012**, *30*, 132–138. [CrossRef]
17. Vrdoljak, J.; Dobranić, V.; Filipović, I.; Zdolec, N. Microbiological quality of soft, semi-hard and hard cheeses during the shelf-life. *Maced. Vet. Rev.* **2016**, *39*, 59–64. [CrossRef]
18. Tittarelli, F.; Perpetuini, G.; Di Gianvito, P.; Tofalo, R. Biogenic amines producing and degrading bacteria: A snapshot from raw ewes' cheese. *LWT Food Sci. Technol.* **2019**, *101*, 1–9. [CrossRef]
19. Zdolec, N.; Bogdanović, T.; Pažin, V.; Šimunić-Mežnarić, V.; Martinec, N.; Lorenzo, J. Control of biogenic amines in dry sausages inoculated with dairy-originated bacteriocinogenic *Enterococcus faecalis* EF-101. *Vet. Arh.* **2020**, *90*, 77–85. [CrossRef]
20. Eerola, S.; Hinkkanen, R.; Lindfors, E.; Hirvi, T. Liquid chromatographic determination of biogenic amines in dry sausages. *J. AOAC Int.* **1993**, *76*, 575–578. [CrossRef]
21. Fox, P.F.; Guinee, T.P.; Cogan, T.M.; McSweeney, P.L.H. Microbiology of cheese ripening. In *Fundamentals of Cheese Science*; Springer: Boston, MA, USA, 2017; pp. 333–390.
22. Ladero, V.; Sanchez-Llana, E.; Fernández, M.; Alvarez, M.A. Survival of biogenic amine-producing dairy LAB strains at pasteurisation conditions. *Int. J. Food Sci. Technol.* **2011**, *46*, 516–521. [CrossRef]
23. Zdolec, N.; Kiš, M. Antimicrobial properties of food enterococci. In *Microbial Biotechnology in Food and Health*; Ray, R.C., Ed.; Academic Press/Elsevier: London, UK, 2021; in press.

24. Franz, C.M.A.P.; Holzapfel, W. The genus Enterococcus: Biotechnological and safety issues. In *Lactic Acid Bacteria: Microbiological and Functional Aspects*, 3rd ed.; Saminen, S., von Wright, O.A., Eds.; Marcel Dekker: New York, NY, USA, 2011; pp. 199–248.
25. Dobranić, V.; Zdolec, N.; Račić, I.; Vujnović, A.; Zdelar-Tuk, M.; Filipović, I.; Grgurević, N.; Špičić, S. Determination of enterotoxin genes in coagulase- negative staphylococci from autochthonous Croatian fermented sausages. *Vet. Arh.* **2013**, *83*, 145–152.
26. Zdolec, N.; Dobranić, V.; Zdolec, G.; Đuričić, D. Antimicrobial resistance of coagulase-negative staphylococci and lactic acid bacteria from industrially produced dairy products. *Mljekarstvo* **2013**, *63*, 30–35.
27. Novella-Rodríguez, S.; Veciana-Nogués, M.T.; Izquierdo-Pulido, M.; Vidal-Carou, M.C. Distribution of biogenic amines and polyamines in cheese. *J. Food Sci.* **2003**, *68*, 750–755. [CrossRef]
28. Komprda, T.; Burdychová, R.; Dohnal, V.; Cwikova, O.; Sládková, P. Some factors influencing biogenic amines and polyamines content in Dutch-type semi-hard cheese. *Eur. Food Res. Technol.* **2007**, *227*, 29–36. [CrossRef]
29. Shalaby, M.A.; Kassem, M.A.; Morsy, O.; Mohamed, N.M. Anti-tyramine potential of *Lactobacillus rhamnosus* (LGG®) in cheese samples collected from Alexandria, Egypt. *Food Biotechnol.* **2020**, *34*, 243–261. [CrossRef]
30. EFSA. Scientific opinion on risk based control of biogenic amine formation in fermented foods. *EFSA J.* **2011**, *9*, 2393. [CrossRef]
31. Buňka, F.; Zálešáková, L.; Flasarová, R.; Pachlová, V.; Budinský, P.; Buňková, L. Biogenic amines content in selected commercial fermented products of animal origin. *J. Microbiol. Biotechnol. Food Sci.* **2012**, *2*, 209–218.
32. Poveda, J.M.; Chicon, R.; Cabezas, L. Biogenic amine content and proteolysis in Manchego cheese manufactured with Lactobacillus paracasei subsp. paracasei as adjunct and other autochthonous strains as starters. *Int. Dairy J.* **2015**, *47*, 94–101. [CrossRef]
33. Renes, E.; Ladero, V.; Tornadijo, M.E.; Fresno, J.M. Production of sheep milk cheese with high γ-aminobutyric acid and ornithine concentration and with reduced biogenic amines level using autochthonous lactic acid bacteria strains. *Food Microbiol.* **2019**, *78*, 1–10. [CrossRef]
34. Barbieri, F.; Montanari, C.; Gardini, F.; Tabanelli, G. Biogenic amine production by lactic acid bacteria: A review. *Foods* **2019**, *8*, 17. [CrossRef]
35. Dobranić, V.; Kazazić, S.; Filipović, I.; Mikulec, N.; Zdolec, N. Composition of raw cow's milk microbiota and identification of enterococci by MALDI-TOF MS-short communication. *Vet. Arh.* **2016**, *86*, 581–590.

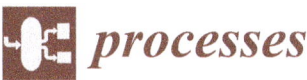

Communication

Microbiome Associated with Slovak Traditional Ewe's Milk Lump Cheese

Andrea Lauková [1,*], Lenka Micenková [2], Monika Pogány Simonová [1], Valentína Focková [1], Jana Ščerbová [1], Martin Tomáška [3], Emília Dvorožňáková [4] and MiroslavOlošta [3]

1. Institute of Animal Physiology, Centre of Biosciences of the Slovak Academy of Sciences, Šoltésovej 4-6, 040 01 Košice, Slovakia; simonova@saske.sk (M.P.S.); fockova@saske.sk (V.F.); scerbova@saske.sk (J.Š.)
2. RECETOX, Faculty of Science, Masaryk University, Kamenice 5, 625 00 Brno, Czech Republic; micenkova@recetox.muni.cz
3. Research Dairy Institute, a.s. Dlhá 95, 010 00 Žilina, Slovakia; martin.tomaska@vumza.sk (M.T.); miroslav.kolosta@vumza.sk (M.K.)
4. Parasitological Institute of the Slovak Academy of Sciences, Šoltésovej 4-6, 040 01 Košice, Slovakia; dvoroz@saske.sk
* Correspondence: laukova@saske.sk; Tel.: +421-557-922-964; Fax: +421-557-827-842

Abstract: Worldwide consumers increasingly demand traditional/local products, to which those made from ewe's milk belong. In Slovakia, dairy products made from ewe's milk have a long tradition. A total of seventeen farmhouse fresh ewe's milk lump cheeses from various local farm producers in central Slovakia were sampled at farms and then analyzed. Based on the sequencing data analysis, the phylum Firmicutes dominated (60.92%) in ewe's lump cheeses, followed with the phylum Proteobacteria (38.23%), Actinobacteria (0.38%) and Bacteroidetes (0.35%). The phylum Firmicutes was represented by six genera, among which the highest amount possessed the genus *Streptococcus* (41.13%) followed with the genus *Lactococcus* (8.54%), *Fructobacillus* (3.91%), *Enterococcus* (3.18%), *Staphylococcus* (1.80%) and the genus *Brochotrix* (0.08%). The phylum Proteobacteria in ewe's lump cheeses involved eight Gram-negative genera: *Pseudomonas*, *Acinetobacter*, *Enterobacter*, *Ewingella*, *Escherichia-Shigella*, *Pantoea* and *Moraxella*. The phylum Bacteroidetes involved three genera: *Bacteroides*, *Sphingobacterium* and *Chrysobacterium*. Results presented are original; the microbiome of Slovak ewe's milk lump cheese has been not analyzed at those taxonomic levels up to now.

Keywords: ewe; milk lump cheese; microbiome

Citation: Lauková, A.; Micenková, L.; Pogány Simonová, M.; Focková, V.; Ščerbová, J.; Tomáška, M.; Dvorožňáková, E.;Ološta, M. Microbiome Associated with Slovak Traditional Ewe's Milk Lump Cheese. *Processes* **2021**, *9*, 1603. https://doi.org/10.3390/pr9091603

Academic Editors: Nevijo Zdolec and Wei Ma

Received: 8 June 2021
Accepted: 6 September 2021
Published: 7 September 2021

Publisher's Note: MDPI stays neutral with regard to jurisdictional claims in published maps and institutional affiliations.

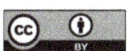

Copyright: © 2021 by the authors. Licensee MDPI, Basel, Switzerland. This article is an open access article distributed under the terms and conditions of the Creative Commons Attribution (CC BY) license (https://creativecommons.org/licenses/by/4.0/).

1. Introduction

Nowadays, consumers increasingly demand traditional products made from ewe's milk. Milk from farm animals and dairy products is a highly nutritious food [1,2], a staple component of human nutrition. However, food safety has become an issue of intensive interest worldwide. Eminent attention is focused on the microbial population in those products. This is because bacteria can show their beneficial potential (production of bacteriocins, probiotic character) but, on the other hand, damaging potential (virulence factor genes presence, drug-resistant genes, etc.), which can threaten human health. Therefore, understanding of the microbiome of products provides information potential for basic science on one hand; on the other hand, it provides information for consumers. It is also a signal to researchers and producers to research how to prevent/avoid/reduce contamination.

In Slovakia, dairy products made from ewe's milk include, e.g., traditional cheeses such as "parenica", "korbáčik" "oštiepok", and Liptauer bryndza, and also ewe's milk lump cheese, either fresh or smoked [3–5]. "Parenica", "korbáčik" "oštiepok" and Liptauer bryndza, as well as Oravian korbáčik cheese and Zázrivá korbáčik cheese, were designed to be PGI products, meaning products with protected geographical indication [6,7]. Fresh ewe's milk lump cheese has been given the TSG label since November 2010, meaning traditional speciality guaranteed [7]. Processing of fresh soft ewe's milk lump cheese consists of the several phases, described in detail in the previous study [4]. This cheese derives its characteristic taste as a result of the traditional technology used during its fermentation and from being shaped by hand into a lump [6]. In general, cheese as a product has a diverse microbial community, which indeed can vary within the cheese from the core to the surface, which is greatly influenced by manufacturing conditions, including ripening conditions. Understanding the composition of this community (microbiota), and its impact on the quality and safety of cheese products, is of critical importance. In addition to, in the majority of cases, consciously added starter and adjunct bacteria (which are added as a supplement), cheese contains a heterogeneous variety of other, non-starter, microorganisms. These various microbiota can play vital roles in the development of the organoleptic properties of cheese, nutrient composition, shelf-life, and safety [8]. The bacterial population in those cheeses has been already studied [2,5] using the standard microbiological method.

However, information describing the microbiome of Slovak ewe's milk lump cheeses analyzed by next-generation sequencing has not been reported up to now. Therefore, the aim of this study was to analyze the microbiome of local ewe's milk lump cheeses using the formerly mentioned sequencing technique.

2. Materials and Methods

A total of seventeen farmhouse fresh ewe's milk lump cheeses from local farm producers in central Slovakia were sampled at farms and transported in our laboratory. After being transported to the laboratory in a refrigerating box, the appropriate volume (100 g) of samples was frozen until further analyses. Individual samples of cheeses were marked as OS1, OS4, OS6, OS8, OS9, OS10, OS11, OS13, OS14, OS15, OS17, OS19, OS51, OS54, OS80, OS94, and OSun following different producers (Figure 1). The appropriate amount of each farmhouse fresh ewe's milk lump soft cheese was homogenized (Stomacher, Masticator, IUL Instruments, Barcelona, Spain). A total of 260 µL of homogenized cheese sample was transferred into 2 mL tubes and 750 µL of bead solution and 60 µL of C1 (kit DNeasy PowerLyzer buffer, QIAGEN, Hilden, Germany) were added to each sample. Next, the total volume was transferred to the bead tubes, and DNA isolation was performed using a DNeasy PowerLyzer PowerSoil Kit (QIAGEN, Hilden, Germany) according to the manufacturer's protocol. Isolated DNA was used as a template in PCR reaction (targeting the hypervariable V4 region of the bacterial 16S rRNA gene according to the 16S Metagenomic Sequencing Library Preparation protocol (Illumina, San Diego, CA, USA). The PCR detection protocol and reagents are shown in Table S1. The primer pairs used are listed in Table 1. Sequencing was performed using MiSeq reagents Kits v2 on a MiSeq 2000 sequencer according to the manufacturers' instructions (Illumina, San Diego, CA, USA).

Table 1. List of primers.

EMP16S-1	F	TCGTCGGCAGCGTCAGATGTGTATAAGAGACAGAGCCTTCGTCGCGTGTGYCAGCMGCCGCGGTAA	
	R	GTCTCGTGGGCTCGGAGATGTGTATAAGAGACAGCCTAACGGTCCACCGGACTACNVGGGTWTCTAAT	
EMP16S-2	F	TCGTCGGCAGCGTCAGATGTGTATAAGAGACAGTCCATACCGGAAGTGTGYCAGCMGCCGCGGTAA	
	R	GTCTCGTGGGCTCGGAGATGTGTATAAGAGACAGCGCGCCTTAAACCCGGACTACNVGGGTWTCTAAT	
EMP16S-3	F	TCGTCGGCAGCGTCAGATGTGTATAAGAGACAGCCCTGCTACAGTGTGYCAGCMGCCGCGGTAA	
	R	GTCTCGTGGGCTCGGAGATGTGTATAAGAGACAGTATGGTACCCAGCCGGACTACNVGGGTWTCTAAT	
EMP16S-4	F	TCGTCGGCAGCGTCAGATGTGTATAAGAGACAGTGAGACCCTACAGTGTGYCAGCMGCCGCGGTAA	
	R	GTCTCGTGGGCTCGGAGATGTGTATAAGAGACAGGCCTCTACGTCGCCGGACTACNVGGGTWTCTAAT	
EMP16S-5	F	TCGTCGGCAGCGTCAGATGTGTATAAGAGACAGACTTGGTGTAAGGTGTGYCAGCMGCCGCGGTAA	16S Metagenomic sequencing
	R	GTCTCGTGGGCTCGGAGATGTGTATAAGAGACAGACTACTGAGGATCCCGGACTACNVGGGTWTCTAAT	Library
EMP16S-6	F	TCGTCGGCAGCGTCAGATGTGTATAAGAGACAGATTACGTATCATGTGTGYCAGCMGCCGCGGTAA	Preparation protocol; Illumina,
	R	GTCTCGTGGGCTCGGAGATGTGTATAAGAGACAGAATTCACCTTCCTCCGGACTACNVGGGTWTCTAAT	San Diego, CA, USA
EMP16S-7	F	TCGTCGGCAGCGTCAGATGTGTATAAGAGACAGCACGCAGTCTACGTGTGYCAGCMGCCGCGGTAA	(EMP 515-806)
	R	GTCTCGTGGGCTCGGAGATGTGTATAAGAGACAGCGCTATAAATGCGCCGGACTACNVGGGTWTCTAAT	
EMP16S-8	F	TCGTCGGCAGCGTCAGATGTGTATAAGAGACAGTGTGCACGCCATGTGTGYCAGCMGCCGCGGTAA	
	R	GTCTCGTGGGCTCGGAGATGTGTATAAGAGACAGATGCTGCAACACCCGGACTACNVGGGTWTCTAAT	
EMP16S-9	F	TCGTCGGCAGCGTCAGATGTGTATAAGAGACAGCCGGACAAGAAGGTGTGYCAGCMGCCGCGGTAA	
	R	GTCTCGTGGGCTCGGAGATGTGTATAAGAGACAGACTCGCTCGTCCCGGACTACNVGGGTWTCTAAT	
EMP16S-10	F	TCGTCGGCAGCGTCAGATGTGTATAAGAGACAGTTGCTGGACGCTGTGTGYCAGCMGCCGCGGTAA	
	R	GTCTCGTGGGCTCGGAGATGTGTATAAGAGACAGTTCCTTAGTAGTCCGGACTACNVGGGTWTCTAAT	
EMP16S-11	F	TCGTCGGCAGCGTCAGATGTGTATAAGAGACAGTACTAACGCGGTGTGTGYCAGCMGCCGCGGTAA	
	R	GTCTCGTGGGCTCGGAGATGTGTATAAGAGACAGCGTCCGTATGAACCGGACTACNVGGGTWTCTAAT	

Table 1. Cont.

EMP16S-12	F	TCGTCGGCAGCGTCAGATGTGTATAAGAGACAGGCGATCACACCTGTGTGYCAGCMGCCGCGGTAA
	R	GTCTCGTGGGCTCGGAGATGTGTATAAGAGACAGACGTGAGGAACGCCGGACTACNVGGGTWTCTAAT
EMP16S-13	F	TCGTCGGCAGCGTCAGATGTGTATAAGAGACAGCAAACGCACTAAGTGTGYCAGCMGCCGCGGTAA
	R	GTCTCGTGGGCTCGGAGATGTGTATAAGAGACAGGGTTGCCCTGTACCGGACTACNVGGGTWTCTAAT
EMP16S-14	F	TCGTCGGCAGCGTCAGATGTGTATAAGAGACAGGAAGAGGGTTGAGTGTGYCAGCMGCCGCGGTAA
	R	GTCTCGTGGGCTCGGAGATGTGTATAAGAGACAGCATATAGCCCGACCGGACTACNVGGGTWTCTAAT
EMP16S-15	F	TCGTCGGCAGCGTCAGATGTGTATAAGAGACAGTGAGTGGTCTGTGTGTGYCAGCMGCCGCGGTAA
	R	GTCTCGTGGGCTCGGAGATGTGTATAAGAGACAGGCCTATGAGATCCCGGACTACNVGGGTWTCTAAT

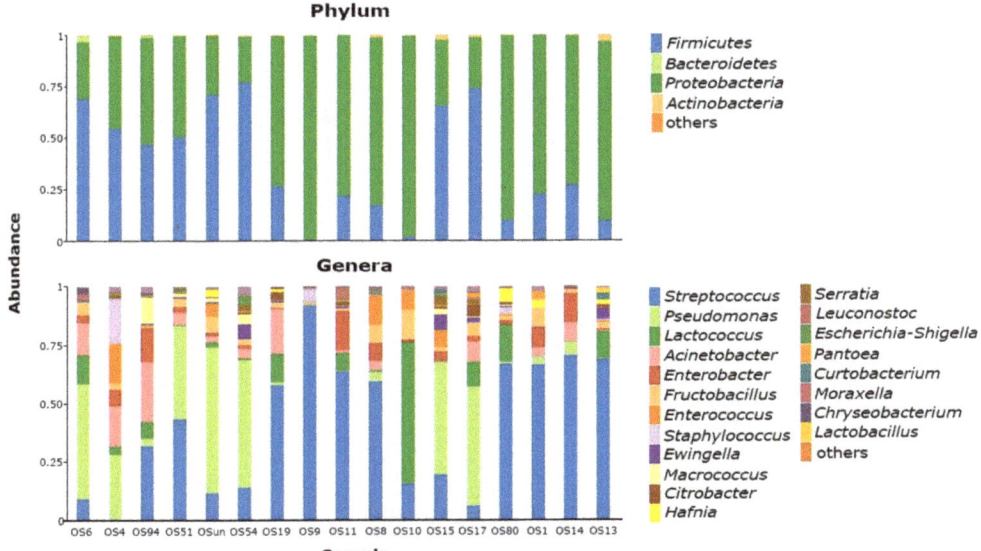

Figure 1. Detection of microbiota at the levels of phyla and genera (individual cheeses are also indicated in Section 2).

Sequence pre-processing included quality trimming using a Trimmomatic sequence tool [9], subsequent joining by the fastq-join utility [10], and demultiplexing. In the final step, joined reads were subjected to operational taxonomic unit (OTU) picking with a 97% sequence similarity threshold. OTU picking was performed using the tool uclust [11]. OTU picking was followed by taxonomy assignment using the usearch-based [11] method of the QIIME 1.9.1 [12] toolset against the Siva v 123 16S rRNA database [13].

3. Results and Discussion

Based on sequencing data, the phylum Firmicutes dominated (60. 92%) in ewe's milk lump cheeses, followed by the phylum Proteobacteria (38. 23%, Table 2 and Figure 2). The other phyla were detected in slight amounts: Actinobacteria (0.38%) and Bacteroidetes (0.35%, Table 2 and Figure 2). The phylum Firmicutes was represented by six (6) involved genera (Figure 3), among which the highest amount possessed the genus *Streptococcus* (41.13%). This genus belongs to the class Bacilli, the order Lactobacillales and to the family Streptococcaceae. Regarding individual cheeses, the OS9 cheese possessed the highest percentage amount of streptococci, while the lowest amount was detected in the cheese OS17 (Figure 1). The cheese OS4 was even streptococci absent. Streptococci are helpful bacteria and their different occurrences in individual cheeses can be influenced by their amount in ewe's milk. The second most frequently detected genus in Slovak traditional ewe's milk lump cheeses was the genus *Lactococcus* (8.54%, Figures 1 and 3). However, its amount was much lower compared with the genus *Streptococcus* (Figures 1 and 3, Table 2). The genus *Lactococcus* also belongs to the class Bacilli and the order Lactobacillales. The genus *Fructobacillus* was the third most frequently occurring microbial representative in ewe's milk lump cheeses (3.91%, Figures 1 and 3), belonging again to the same class and order, but to the family Leuconostocacae [14]. The detection of lactobacilli and leuconostoc was very slight in the individual ewe's lump cheeses (Figures 1 and 3). However, those formerly mentioned genera belong to helpful/beneficial microbiota in milk, e.g., representatives of the genera *Streptococcus, Leuconostoc* or *Lactobacillus* are able to utilize lactose which is broken down in the lactic acid [1]. Streptococci, lactococci and lactobacilli belong to Gram-positive bacteria which can be commonly detected in cheeses, especially in those produced with starter cultures [15]. The genus *Enterococcus* belonging in the family Enterococcacae was detected in tested cheeses in the amount of 3.18% (Figures 1 and 3). On the one hand, enterococci can be supposed to be contaminant bacteria in cheeses [16–18]; on the other hand, they can serve as probiotic microbiota producing antimicrobial active substances—bacteriocins [2,19]. However, representatives of the genus *Staphylococcus* are supposed to be frequent inhabitants in cheeses [4,20]. They were detected in ewe's lump cheese in the amount of 1.80% (Table 2, Figures 1 and 3). However, helpful/beneficial microbiota can also cause some technological changes when they are over-produced [2], so their optimal amount is preferred. The genus *Brochotrix* belonging to the family Listeriacae was evaluated in cheeses in very slight amounts (0.08%).

Table 2. Abundance percentage (%) in the microbiome analyses of ewe's milk lump cheese.

Phylum			
Firmicutes (60.92)	Proteobacteria (38.23)	Actinobacteria (0.38)	Bacteroidetes (0.35)
Genera			
Streptococcus (41.13)	*Pseudomonas* (20.70)	*Curtobacterium* (0.7%)	*Chryseobacterium* (0.03)
Lactococcus (8.54)	*Acinetobacter* (6.79)		*Shingobacterium* (0.03)
Fructobacillus (3.91)	*Enterobacter* (5.14)		*Bacteroides* (0.001)
Enterococcus (3.18)	*Ewingella* (1.3)		
Staphylococcus (1.80)	*Escherichia-Shigella* (0.55)		
Brochotrix (0.08)	*Pantoea* (0.46)		
	Moraxella (0.31)		

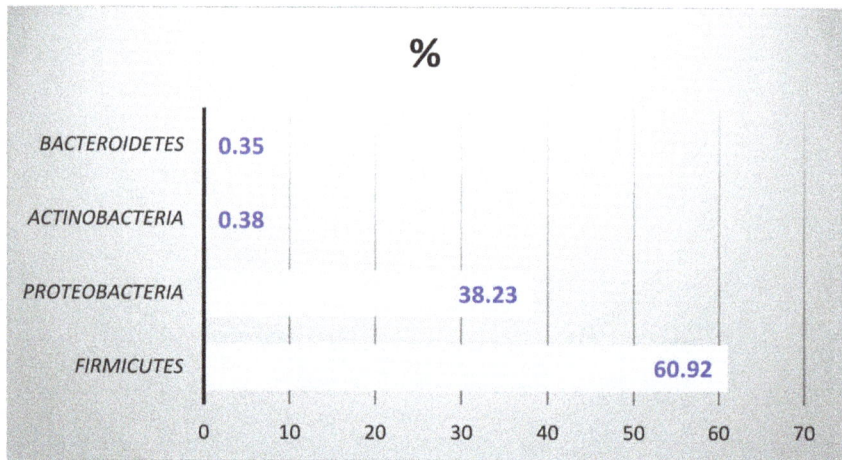

Figure 2. Phyla detected in Slovak ewe's lump cheeses (in percentage).

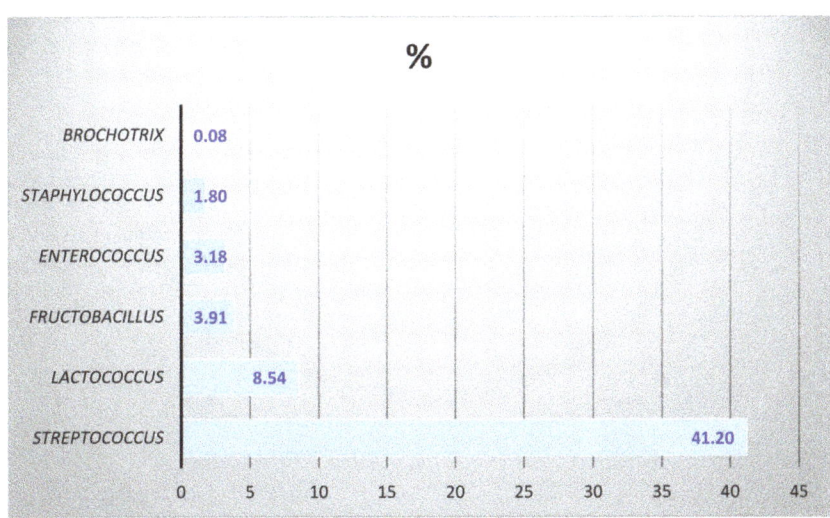

Figure 3. Gram-positive genera detected in Slovak ewe's lump cheeses (in percentage).

However, spoilage bacterial phyla were also detected in analyzed cheeses. The phylum Proteobacteria detected in ewe's milk lump cheeses was represented by eight (8) Gram-negative genera: *Pseudomonas, Acinetobacter, Enterobacter, Ewingella, Escherichia-Shigella, Pantoea* and *Moraxella*. Regarding the phylum Proteobacteria, surprisingly, the genus *Pseudomonas* (20.7%) was evaluated in the highest amount (Table 2, Figures 1 and 4) followed by the genera *Acinetobacter* (6.79%), *Enterobacter* (5.14%), *Ewingella* (1.3%), *Escherichia-Shigella* (0.55%), *Pantoea* (0.46%) and *Moraxella* (0.31%, Figures 1 and 4, Table 2). In the phylum Actinobacteria the genus *Curtobacterium* was evaluated, belonging to the order Actinomycetales/Micrococcales and the family Microbacteriacae [21]. The highest amount of pseudomonads was determined in the cheese OSun, OS6 and OS54 (Figures 1 and 4); on the other hand, in the cheeses OS9 and OS11, these bacteria were not found. Psychrotrophic microbiota such as pseudomonads are able to grow at low temperatures; this can explain their occurrence in cheeses. *Pseudomonas* spp. can enter cheese, e.g., via water. They produce enzymes which tolerate low temperatures and break down proteins in products. This leads to organoleptic changes. The presence of harmful bacteria can also indicate insufficient hygiene conditions during the manufacturing of cheeses. However, the quality of this type of cheeses can be influenced by external factors, such as the temperature during transportation, the quality of milk, the animals' location, etc. Even in spite of sufficient sanitary condition maintenance, Gram-negative bacteria as well as unfavorable Gram-positive bacteria can contaminate cheeses [22,23]. From those Gram-positive, e.g., representatives of the genus *Brochotrix* can appear as a consequence of temperature imbalance. However, in ewe's milk lump cheeses, listeriae were not detected. Kačániová et al. [24] reported representatives of the genera *Escherichia, Acinetobacter* and *Enterobacter* detected in Liptauer bryndza using the standard microbial technique.

The microbiome in traditional/local farmhouse ewe's milk lump cheeses is a variable community. Gram-positive bacterial genera in fresh ewe's milk lump cheeses are associated with natural occurrence. Commonly, lactic acid bacteria (LAB) are a dominant population in raw milk [25]. Additionally, in the microbiome of ewe's milk lump cheeses, genera belonging to LAB (*Lactococcus, Streptococcus* and/or *Enterococcus*) were detected. Salazar et al. [26] used the sequencing method to determine the microbial community associated with Gouda cheese. Based on the percentage of sequence reads, they similarly found the genera *Lactococcus, Streptococcus, Staphylococcus* and *Lactobacillus* to be dominant organisms in cheese. Kačániová et al. [24] detected lactococci and staphylococci in traditional Liptauer bryndza, which is made from ewe's milk lump cheese. Enterococci are commonly found in high levels in a variety of cheeses produced from raw ewe's milk [27,28]. Different species of enterococci isolated from cheeses were able to produce antimicrobial peptides—enterocins [29]; most of them also showed probiotic character [24]. Altogether, this indicates their benefit in the products. Despite the fact that in the ewe's milk lump cheeses tested, the genus *Streptococcus* was detected in high amounts, no information exists about species representatives in cheese in the literature. In May bryndza cheese, again, only *Streptococcus* spp. was reported [24]. Plaský et al. [30] used metagenomic analysis for Slovak bryndza cheese produced in winter containing ewe's milk lump cheese. They detected a diverse prokaryotic microbiota composed mostly of the genera *Lactococcus*, *Streptococcus*, *Lactobacillus* and *Enterococcus*. They also detected some Gammaproteobacteria. This indicates a similar composition of cheeses made from ewe's milk.

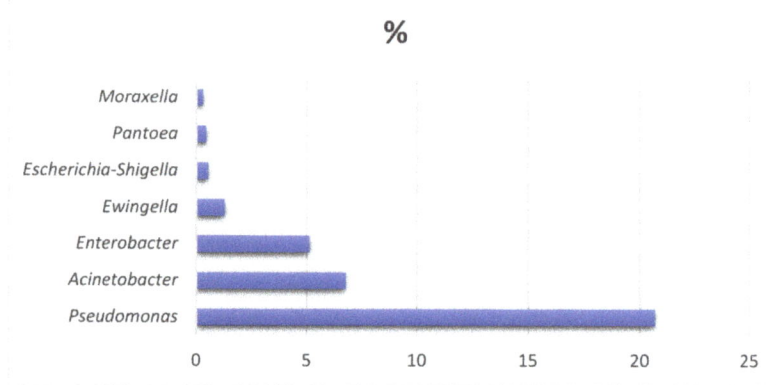

Figure 4. Gram-negative genera detected in Slovak ewe's lump cheese (in percentage).

4. Conclusions

The sequencing method allows for microbial consortia in ewe's milk lump cheese to be determined more accurately and shows how the microbiome plays a role in safety and quality. It can be seen that fresh lump cheeses possess many beneficial and non-useful microbiota; however, the phylum Firmicutes and the genus *Streptococcus* dominate.

Supplementary Materials: The following is available online at https://www.mdpi.com/article/10.3390/pr9091603/s1. It is available in Table S1. The PCR protocol and reagents used in bacterial analysis of ewe's milk lump cheeses.

Author Contributions: Conceptualization, designing, summarizing, writing, project administration; A.L. methodology, sequencing L.M.; investigation, M.P.S., V.F. and J.Š. resources, M.T., M.K. and E.D. All authors have read and agreed to the published version of the manuscript.

Funding: This research was funded by the Slovak Research and Development Agency under contract no. APVV-17-0028 and the RECETOX research infrastructure: the Czech Ministry of Education, Youth and Sports (LM2018121,02.1.01/0.0/0.0/18_046/0015975, and CZ.02.1.01/0.0/0.0/16013/0001761.

Institutional Review Board Statement: Not applicable.

Informed Consent Statement: Not applicable.

Data Availability Statement: Data availability regarding the PCR are in Supplementary Materials Table S1.

Acknowledgments: We are grateful for language editing Andrew Billingham.

Conflicts of Interest: The authors declare no conflict of interest.

References

1. Uhrín, V.; Lauková, A.; Jančová, A.; Plintovič, V. *Mlieko a Mliečna Žľaza. Milk and Mammary Gland*; Publ. No. 92; Faculty of Natural Sciences of the University Constantinus Philosophus: Nitra, Slovakia, 2002; pp. 5–167, ISBN 80-8050-511-X. (in Slovak)
2. Lauková, A.; Focková, V.; Simonová, M.P. *Enterococcus mundtii* Isolated from Slovak Raw Goat Milk and Its Bacteriocinogenic Potential. *Int. J. Environ. Res. Public Health* **2020**, *17*, 9504. [CrossRef]
3. Herian. Benefit of sheep milk products to human health. *Milk Lett. Mlékařské Listy* **2014**, *143*, 1–6. (In Slovak)
4. Lauková, A.; Simonová, M.P.; Focková, V.; Košta, M.; Tomáška, M.; Dvorožňáková, E. Susceptibility to Bacteriocins in Biofilm-Forming, Variable Staphylococci Isolated from Local Ewe's Milk Lump Cheeses. *Foods* **2020**, *9*, 1335. [CrossRef] [PubMed]
5. Vatačšinová, T.; Pipová, M.; Fraqueza, M.J.R.; Maľa, P.; Dudríková, E.; Drážovská, M.; Lauková, A. Short communication: Antimicrobial Potential of *Lactobacillus plantarum* Strains Isolated from Slovak Raw Sheep Milk Cheeses. *J. Dairy Sci.* **2020**, *103*, 6900–6903. [CrossRef] [PubMed]
6. Supeková, S.; Honza, M.; Kačenová, D. Perception of Slovak Foodstuffs Designated by Protected Geographical Indication by Slovak Consumers. *J. Food Nutr. Res.* **2008**, *47*, 205–208.
7. The Slovak Spectator. 2011. Available online: https://spectator.sme.sk (accessed on 6 August 2021).
8. Fox, P.F.; McSweeney, P.L.H.; Cogan, T.M.; Guinee, T.P. *Fundamentals of Cheese Science*, 4th ed.; Springer: Boston, MA, USA, 2017; pp. 185–229. ISBN 978-0-8342-1260-2.
9. Bolger, A.M.; Lohse, M.; Usadel, B. Trimmomatic: A Flexible Trimmer for Illumina Sequence Data. *Bioinformatics* **2014**, *30*, 2114–2120. [CrossRef] [PubMed]
10. Aronesty, E. Ea-utils. "Command-Line Tools for Processing Biological Sequencing Data". Available online: https://github.com/ExpressionAnalysis/ea-utils (accessed on 20 June 2020).
11. Edgar, R.C. Search and clustering orders of magnitude faster than BLAST. *Bioinformatics* **2010**, *26*, 2460–2461. [CrossRef]
12. Caporaso, J.G.; Kuczynski, J.; Stombaugh, J.; Bittinger, K.; Bushman, F.D.; Costello, E.K.; Fierer, N.; Peña, A.G.; Goodrich, J.K.; Gordon, J.I.; et al. QIIME allows analysis of high-throughput community sequencing data. *Nat. Meth.* **2010**, *7*, 335–336. [CrossRef]
13. Quast, C.; Pruesse, E.; Yilmaz, P.; Gerken, J.; Schweer, T.; Yarza, P.; Peplies, J.; Glockner, F.O. The SILVA ribosomal RNA gene database project: Improved data processing and web-based tools. *Nucl. Acids Res.* **2013**, *41*, D590–D596. [CrossRef]
14. Endo, A.; Dicks, L.M.T. *Lactic Acid Bacteria: Biodiversity and Taxonomy*; Holzapfel, W.H., Wood, B.J.B., Eds.; Wiley-Blackwell: Hoboken, NJ, USA, 2014; p. 632, ISBN 9781444333831.
15. Bouton, Y.; Buchin, S.; Duboz, G.; Pochet, S.; Beuvier, E. Effect of mesophilic lactobacilli and enterococci adjunct cultures on the final characteristics of a microfiltered milk Swiss-type cheese. *Food Microbiol.* **2009**, *26*, 183–191. [CrossRef]
16. Tofalo, R.; Schirone, M.; Fasoli, G.; Perpetuini, G.; Patrignani, F.; Manetta, A.C.; Lanciotti, R.; Corsetti, A.; Martino, G.; Suzzi, G. Influence of pig rennet on proteolysis, organic acids content and microbiota of Pecorino di Farindola, a traditional Italian ewe's raw milk cheese. *Food Chem.* **2015**, *175*, 121–127. [CrossRef] [PubMed]
17. Tofalo, R.; Perpetuini, G.; Battistelli, N.; Pepe, A.; Ianni, A.; Martino, G.; Suzzi, G. Accumulation γ-Aminobutyric Acid and Biogenic Amines in a Traditional Raw Milk Ewe's Cheese. *Foods* **2019**, *8*, 401. [CrossRef]
18. Tsanasidou, C.; Asimakoula, S.; Sameli, N.; Fanitsios, C.; Vandera, E.; Bosnea, L.; Koukkou, A.-I.; Samelis, J. Safety Evaluation, Biogenic Amine Formation, and Enzymatic Activity Profiles of Autochthonous Enterocin-Producing Greek Cheese Isolates of the *Enterococcus faecium/durans* Group. *Microorganisms* **2021**, *9*, 777. [CrossRef]
19. Franz, C.M.A.P.; Huch, M.; Abriouel, H.; Holzapfel, W.; Gálvez, A. Enterococci as probiotics and their implications in food safety. *Int. J. Food Microbiol.* **2011**, *151*, 125–140. [CrossRef] [PubMed]
20. Issa, G.; Aksu, H. Detection of Methicillin-Resistant *Staphylococcus aureus* in Milk by PCR-Based Phenotyping and Genotyping. *Acta Veterinaria Eurasia* **2020**, *46*, 120–124. [CrossRef]
21. Chase, A.B.; Arevalo, P.; Polz, M.F.; Berlemont, R.; Martiny, J.B.H. Evidence for Ecological Flexibility in the Cosmopolitan Genus *Curtobacterium*. *Front. Microbiol.* **2016**, *7*, 1874. [CrossRef]
22. Quigley, L.; O'Sullivan, O.; Stanton, C.; Beresford, T.P.; Ross, R.P.; Fitzgerald, G.F.; Cotter, P.D. The complex microbiota of raw milk. *FEMS Microbiol.* **2013**, *37*, 664–698. [CrossRef]
23. Kazeminia, M.; Mahmoudi, R.; Ghajarbeygi, P.; Mousavi, S. The effect of seasonal variation on the chemical and microbial quality of raw milk samples used in Qazvin. *Iran. J. Chem. Health Risk* **2019**, *9*, 157–165.
24. Kačániová, M.; Kunová, S.; Štefániková, J.; Felšociová, S.; Godovčíková, L.; Horská, E.; Nagyová, Ľ.; Haščík, P.; Terentjeva, M. Microbiota of the traditional Slovak sheep cheese "Bryndza". *J. Microbiol. Biotechnol. Food Sci.* **2019**, *9*, 482–486. [CrossRef]
25. Šaková, N.; Sádecká, J.; Lejková, J.; Puškárová, A.; Koreňová, J.; Kolek, E.; Valík, Ľ.; Kuchta, T.; Pangallo, D. Characterization of May bryndza cheese from various regions in Slovakia based on microbial, molecular and principal volatile odorants examinations. *J. Food Nutr. Sci.* **2015**, *54*, 239–251.
26. Salazar, J.K.; Carstens, C.K.; Ramachadran, P.; Shazer, A.G.; Narula, S.S.; Reed, E.; Ottesen, A.; Schill, K.M. Metagenomics of pasteurized and unpasteurized gouda cheese using targeted 16S rDNA sequencing. *BMC Microbiol.* **2018**, *18*, 189. [CrossRef] [PubMed]
27. Gelsomino, R.; Vancanneyt, M.; Condon, S.; Swings, J.; Cogan, T.M. Enterococcal diversity in the environment of an Irish Cheddar-type cheesemaking factory. *Int. J. Food Microbiol.* **2001**, *71*, 177–188. [CrossRef]
28. Lauková, A.; Kandričáková, A.; Bino, E.; Tomáška, M.; Kološta, M.; Kmeť, V.; Strompfová, V. Some safety aspects of enterococci isolated from Slovak lactic acid dairy product "žinčica". *Folia Microbiol.* **2020**, *65*, 79–85. [CrossRef] [PubMed]

29. Foulquié-Moreno, M.R.; Sarantinopoulos, P.; Tsakalidou, E.; De Vuyst, L. The role and application of enterococci in food and health. *Int. J. Food Microbiol.* **2006**, *106*, 1–24. [CrossRef] [PubMed]
30. Plany, M.; Kuchta, T.; Šoltýs, K.; Szemes, T.; Pangallo, D.; Siekel, P. Metagenomics analysis of Slovak bryndza cheese using next-generation 16S rDNA amplicon sequencing. *Nova Biotechnol. Chim.* **2016**, *15*, 23–34. [CrossRef]

Identification of *Penicillium verrucosum*, *Penicillium commune*, and *Penicillium crustosum* Isolated from Chicken Eggs

Soňa Demjanová, Pavlina Jevinová, Monika Pipová * and Ivana Regecová

Department of Food Hygiene, Technology and Safety, The University of Veterinary Medicine and Pharmacy in Košice, Komenského 73, 041 81 Košice, Slovakia; sona.demjanova@student.uvlf.sk (S.D.); pavlina.jevinova@uvlf.sk (P.J.); ivana.regecova@uvlf.sk (I.R.)
* Correspondence: monika.pipova@uvlf.sk

Abstract: *Penicillium* species belong to main causative agents of food spoilage leading to significant economic losses and potential health risk for consumers. These fungi have been isolated from various food matrices, including table eggs. In this study, both conventional Polymerase Chain Reaction (PCR) and Polymerase Chain Reaction-Internal Transcribed Spacer-Restriction Fragment Length Polymorphism (PCR-ITS-RFLP) methods were used for species identification of *Penicillium* (P.) spp. isolated from the eggshells of moldy chicken eggs. Seven restriction endonucleases (*Bsp1286*I, *Xma*I, *Hae*III, *Hinf*I, *Mse*I, *Sfc*I, *Hpy188*I) were applied to create ribosomal restriction patterns of amplified ITS regions. To identify *P. verrucosum*, *P. commune*, and *P. crustosum* with the help of conventional PCR assay, species-specific primer pairs VERF/VERR, COMF/COMR, and CRUF/CRUR were designed on the base of 5.8 subunit-Internal Transcribed Spacer (5.8S-ITS) region. Altogether, 121 strains of microscopic filamentous fungi were isolated by traditional culture mycological examination. After morphological evaluation of both macroscopic and microscopic features, 96 strains were classified in *Penicillium* spp. Two molecular methods used have confirmed eight isolates as *P. verrucosum*, 42 isolates as *P. commune*, and 19 isolates as *P. crustosum*. Both PCR-ITS-RFLP and conventional PCR assays appear to be suitable alternatives for rapid identification of the above mentioned *Penicillium* species.

Keywords: mold; egg; *Penicillium*; colony morphology; Ehrlich reaction; creatine; restriction enzyme; PCR; PCR-ITS-RFLP

1. Introduction

Penicillium spp. is one of the most common microscopic filamentous fungi in food-processing industry with more than 200 species known so far [1]. As mesophiles, *Penicillium* species grow best at temperatures between 5 °C and 37 °C, water activity from 0.78 to 0.88 and pH level from 3 to 4.5. They occur in soil, on decomposing vegetation and compost, on dried food, spices, cereals, in fresh fruits and vegetables, as well as in the air and dust [2]. They can also grow on the building walls, especially when the humidity of building material is high [3]. Many *Penicillium* species have the ability to produce a wide range of metabolites, including antibiotics, antiviral agents, and mycotoxins [4].

Foods of animal origin, and in particular table eggs, are also susceptible to contamination by microscopic filamentous fungi. This contamination can be involved by a variety of sources, e.g., feces, litter, feed, but also from improper handling and storage [5]. In accordance with Commission Regulation No 589/2008 [6], fresh table eggs can be stored at temperatures above +5 °C for 28 days after laying. Such conditions favor the development of molds on the eggshell and often lead to significant economic losses due to egg devaluation and subsequent condemnation. Currently, no information on the occurrence of individual *Penicillium* species in table eggs are available worldwide. Fungal species, including *Penicillium* (P.) *crustosum* and *P. verrucosum*, have already been identified among cheese contaminating mycoflora with reported optimum growth temperatures between 15 °C and 25 °C [7–9]. As temperatures close to +15 °C are preferably used in egg storage facilities, the presence of all the three *Penicillium* species could be predicted in table eggs during storage.

Monitoring and identification of microscopic filamentous fungi in food has gained increased attention of food producers, control authorities, and researchers around the world. Identification of *Penicillium* species is primarily based on morphological criteria, such as macroscopic and microscopic features [10,11]. However, this often leads to identification problems. Classical cultivation methods are time-consuming, labor-intensive, non-quantitative, and susceptible to contamination and inaccuracies in classification.

Rapid and reliable identification of microscopic filamentous fungi can contribute to better process management and control in the food sector as well as to a higher level of consumers' health protection. Therefore, molecular methods focused on genotypic characterization have proved their utility. In general, genomic deoxyribonucleic acid (DNA) analysis using the Polymerase Chain Reaction (PCR)-based methods is a fast, sensitive, and reliable possibility for differentiation of microorganisms [12]. In fungal diagnostics, sequence targets within the ribosomal DNA gene complex are proven in identifying different species of microscopic filamentous fungi. Internal Transcribed Spacer (ITS) sequences of ribosomal ribonucleic acid (rRNA) including the highly conserved 18S, 5.8S, 28S genes and internal transcribed spacer regions ITS1 and ITS show low intraspecific polymorphism and high interspecies variability [13]. Currently, the ITS region amplification and sequencing followed by comparison to sequences deposited in the GenBank is the preferred method worldwide. So far, many molecular techniques have been developed for studying population genetic diversity. Such methods as amplified fragment length polymorphism (AFLP), random amplified polymorphic DNA (RAPD), or mini/microsatellite DNA are used to detect polymorphisms at the genome level. The restriction fragment length polymorphism (RFLP) can be used to distinguish variations in the DNA sequences that may not be expressed at the protein level [14,15].

P. verrucosum, *P. commune*, and *P. crustosum* are frequently reported causes of spoilage in wide range of plant food and food materials [16–18]. Moreover, *P. verrucosum* is known for production of ochratoxin A [19] and citrinin [20], and *P. crustosum* is capable of producing penitrem A [21] and roquefortine C [20]. Production of fumigaclavines A and B [22], penitrem A, roquefortine [23], and cyclopiazonic acid has already been reported for *P. commune* [20].

Morphological identification of the above species is time-consuming, challenging, and often inaccurate in the classification. The aim of this study was to design a rapid and effective identification method for *Penicillium* species isolated from table eggs. So far, conventional PCR assays have not been used to distinguish closely related species of *P. verrucosum*, *P. commune*, and *P. crustosum*. Therefore, three species-specific primer pairs were designed and introduced in this study. To verify the specificity and reliability of the newly designed PCR protocol, the results were confirmed by PCR-ITS-RFLP analysis.

2. Materials and Methods

2.1. Mold Cultures

The strains of microscopic filamentous fungi were isolated from the shell surfaces of 40 moldy chicken eggs from Slovak laying hen breeding according to the instructions of STN ISO 21527-1 [24] and STN ISO 21527-2 [25].

2.2. Phenotypic Identification

Mold isolates were tested phenotypically according to standardized procedures [11]. Isolated colonies of microscopic filamentous fungi considered to belong to different mold genera or species were inoculated on the surface of Yeast Extract Sucrose agar medium (YES), Czapek Yeast Autolysate agar medium (CYA) and Malt Extract Agar medium (MEA) (Hi-Media, Mumbia, India) and incubated for 7 days at 25 °C. Macroscopic evaluation was focused on the rate of colony growth, color, texture and corrugation, and the presence of exudate and pigment. Microscopic evaluation was performed on agar preparations stained with lacto phenol cotton blue under optical microscope. Micromorphological structures (stripes, metulae, phialides, and conidia) were measured and documented using the B-290TB optical microscope and Optika Vision Lite 2.13 analysis software (OPTIKA® Microscopes, Ponteranica, Italy).

All isolates classified in *Penicillium* spp. were identified according to the criteria of Frisvad and Samson [11]. Individual *Penicillium* strains grown on CYA were further tested for the production of cyclopiazonic acid and other alkaloids reacting with Ehrlich reagent. In this test, the violet or purple reaction was considered positive for cyclopiazonic acid production, while the yellow or pink reactions indicated the production of other alkaloids. Negative reaction was not manifested by any change in color. Ability of strains to metabolize creatine with concomitant acid production was determined by inoculation of Creatine Sucrose Agar medium (CREA; Hi-Media, Mumbia, India).

2.3. DNA Isolation

Total genomic DNA of the tested strains was isolated by a two-step procedure using zircon and glass beads, Proteinase K (Macherey-Nagel GmbH & Co., Dueren, Germany), ultrasound waves and commercially available E.Z.N.A.® Fungal DNA Mini Kit (OMEGA Bio-tek, Inc., Norcross, GA, USA) according to Regecová et al. [26]. The purity and concentration of DNA was measured using the BioSpec spectrophotometer (SHIMADZU, Kjóto, Japan).

2.4. Species-Specific Identification by PCR-ITS-RFLP Method

The universal primers ITS1 5′-TCCGTAGGTGAACCTGCGG-3′ (forward) and ITS4 5′-TCCTCCGCTTATTGATATGC-3′ (reverse) were used for amplification of the 5.8S-ITS region in tested isolates [27].

The amplification was performed in a volume of 20 µL containing 4.0 µL HOT Firepol® Blend Master Mix (Solis BioDyne, Tartu, Estonia), 0.5 µL of each primer (concentration 10 pmol/µL) and 1 ng to 10 ng of DNA in the thermal cycler TC-512 (Techne, Stadfforshire, UK). The PCR protocol used was as follows: initial cycling step at 95 °C for 12 min, DNA denaturation at 95 °C for 20 s, annealing at 53 °C for 60 s, and elongation at 72 °C for 2 min. The amplification was terminated by cooling to 6 °C.

The following reference strains were used as positive controls in this study: *P. verrucosum* ATCC® 44407™ (American Type Culture Collection, Manassas, VA, USA), *P. commune* CCM F-327, and *P. crustosum* CCM 8322 (Czech Collection of Microorganisms, Brno, Czech Republic).

The PCR products were subsequently digested with restriction endonucleases *Bsp1286*I, *Xma*I, *Hae*III, *Hinf*I, *Mse*I, *Sfc*I, and *Hpy188*I (New England BioLabs®Inc., Ipswich, MA, USA) by modified procedure according to Diguţă et al. [28]. The length of individual fragments was evaluated using the GelAnalyzer 19.1. (Version 14.0.0.0; Oracle Corporation, Redwood City, CA, USA).

2.5. Species-Specific Identification by Conventional PCR Method

Fungal isolates were also identified by conventional PCR method. The primer design was based on ITS region and 5.8S rRNA sequences available in the GenBank-European molecular Biology Laboratory database (GenBank-EMBL).

The 5.8S-ITS rRNA sequences of *P. verrucosum*, *P. crustosum*, and *P. commune* reference strains were retrieved from available databases (GenBank and EMBL). The primers were designed with the help of Primer3 Input (Version 0.4.0; http://bioinfo.ut.ee/primer3-0.4.0/) and then synthesized commercially by Amplia s.r.o. (Bratislava, Slovakia). These primers were reported to amplify a conserved region of 99 bp of the 18S rRNA gene in all the eukaryotic species [29]. The amplification protocol was similar to that described for PCR-ITS-RFLP method, but the annealing ran at different temperatures depending on the type of primer used (Table 1).

Table 1. Primers designed and used in this study.

Primer Name	Primer Sequence (5′-3′)	Annealing Temperature (°C)	Size of PCR Product	GenBank-EMBL Accession Number
	Penicillium verrucosum			
VERF	TCGTAACAAGGTTTCCGTAGG	59	607 bp	DQ681351.1
VERR	TTTCCTTCCGCCTTATTGAT			
	Penicillium commune			
COMF	CCCGTGTTTATTTTACCTTG	51	464 bp	GQ340555.1
COMR	CTGGATAAAATTTGGGTTGA			
	Penicillium crustosum			
CRUF	TCCCACCCGTGTTTATTTTA	58	892 bp	HQ225711.1
CRUR	TCCCTTTCAACAATTTCACG			

The reference strains used as positive controls in the conventional PCR protocol included *P. verrucosum* ATCC® 44407™ (American Type Culture Collection, Manassas, VA, USA), *P. commune* CCM F-327, *P. crustosum* CCM 8322, *P. chrysogenum* CCM F-362, *P. brevicompactum* CCM 8040, *P. glabrum* CCM F-310, and *P. expansum* CCM F-576 (Czech Collection of Microorganisms, Brno, Czech Republic).

2.6. Detection of PCR Products

The PCR products were size fractionated in agarose gels (1.5%) with the GelRed™Nucleic Acid gel stain (Biotium, Inc., Fremont, CA, USA). Amplicons were visualized by UV transillumination using the Mini Bis Pro® (DNR Bio-Imaging Systems Ltd., Neve Yamin, Izrael). The DNA Ladder of 50 bp (Sigma-Aldrich, Saint Louis, MO, USA) was used as molecular size marker for PCR-ITS-RFLP and the DNA Ladder of 100 bp (Sigma-Aldrich, Saint Louis, MO, USA) was used for species-specific PCR identification.

The identity of PCR products with the selected primers was confirmed by a commercial company (GATC Biotech AG, Cologne, Germany). The DNA sequences obtained from fungal strains were searched for homology to those available at the GenBank-EMBL database using the Basic Local Alignment Search Tool (BLAST) program (NCBI, software package 3.40, Bethesda, MD, USA).

3. Results

3.1. Phenotypic Identification

Strains of microscopic filamentous fungi (n = 121) isolated from chicken eggshells were subjected to phenotypic identification. According to characteristic macroscopic and microscopic features, 96 isolates were identified as *Penicillium* spp. Confirmed isolates were further examined by both Ehrlich reaction and Creatine test. Based on the results obtained, 12 isolates were identified as *P. verrucosum*, 42 as *P. commune*, and 21 as *P. crustosum* (Table 2).

Strains of microscopic filamentous fungi classified as *P. verrucosum* shown a good growth on MEA, CYA, and YES media, with average colony diameters (25.25 ± 8.84) mm for MEA; (25.42 ± 8.56) mm for CYA and (22 ± 10.41) mm for YES agar after 7 day incubation at 25 °C. On both MEA and CYA, colonies were velutinous to floccose texture, green with a white edge hem and corrugation. Clear copious exudate droplets were present. Reverse colony color was light yellow-brown on MEA and cream yellow on CYA. Velutinous green colonies with a white edge hem and beige brown to terracotta reverse color were typical for *P. verrucosum* grown on YES medium. Conidiophores were terverticillate with rough walled-stripe, phialides were cylindrical tapering to a distinct collulum. Conidia were smooth-walled or rough-walled, globose to subglobose. Negative Ehrlich reaction was observed in nine isolates (Table 2, Figure 1).

Table 2. Phenotypic features and morphological identification of three *Penicillium* species isolated from chicken eggs.

Fungal Species	Number of Isolates	Colony Size (mm)			Ehrlich Reaction	Creatine Test	
		MEA	CYA	YES		Growth	Acid Production
Penicillium verrucosum	12	13–37	14–41	11–41	negative (9) pink (2) yellow (1)	weak (7) good (5)	– (8) + (4)
Penicillium commune	48	26–40	23–41	24–42	negative (6) purple (10) violet (32)	weak (9) good (39)	+ (11) ++ (13) +++ (24)
Penicillium crustosum	21	27–37	28–39	24–39	negative (13) yellow (8)	weak (7) good (14)	– (7) ++ (14)

MEA Malt Extract Agar; CYA Czapek Yeast Autolysate agar; YES Yeast Extract Sucrose agar; – none; + weak; ++ good; +++ strong; numbers in parentheses indicate the number of strains showing a particular reaction.

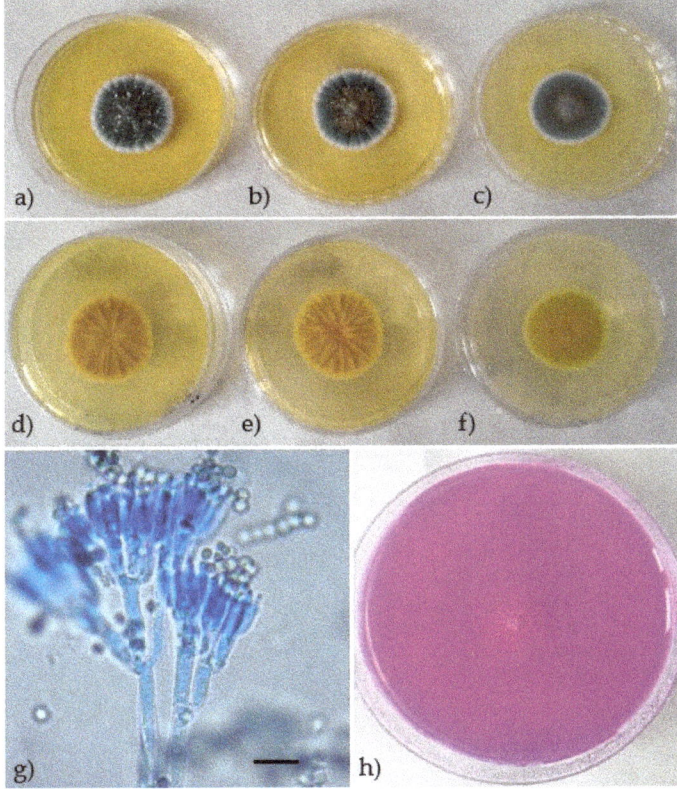

Figure 1. *Penicillium verrucosum*. Seven-day-old colonies on Malt Extract Agar (MEA) (**a**) obverse, (**d**) reverse, Czapek Yeast Autolysate agar (CYA) (**b**) obverse, (**e**) reverse, Yeast Extract Sucrose agar (YES) (**c**) obverse, (**f**) reverse, (**h**) Creatine Sucrose Agar (CREA)—no acid production, (**g**) conidiophores and conidia. Scale: black bar = 10 µm.

The growth of *P. commune* isolates on MEA, CYA, and YES media was very good with average colony diameters (35.46 ± 3.78) mm for MEA, (35.46 ± 4.45) mm for CYA and (33.63 ± 5.30) mm for YES agar following incubation at 25 °C for 7 days. Colonies on both MEA and CYA were floccose to fasciculate texture, blue green to green color with a white edge hem. Clear exudate droplets were often observed. Reverse colony color was beige to beige brown on MEA and cream yellow on CYA. Velutinous blue green colonies with a white edge hem, corrugation, and beige yellow reverse color were typical for *P. commune* grown on YES medium. Conidiophores were terverticillate with rough-walled stripe, phialides cylindrical tapering to a distinct collulum. Conidia were smooth-walled, globose to subglobose. The potential production of cyclopiazonic acid was manifested in 32 isolates as violet reaction and in another 10 isolates as purple reaction. In a half of *P. commune* isolates, strong acid production was also confirmed (Table 2, Figure 2).

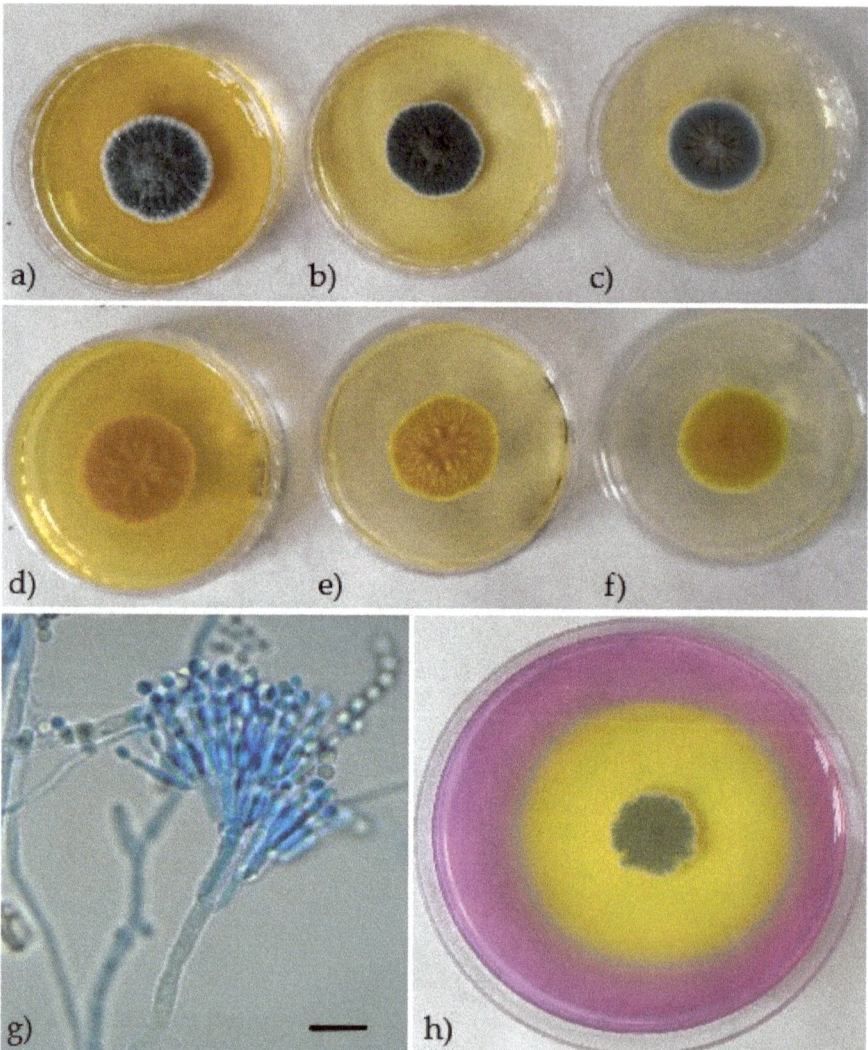

Figure 2. *Penicillium commune*. Seven-day-old colonies on Malt Extract Agar (MEA) (**a**) obverse, (**d**) reverse, Czapek Yeast Autolysate agar (CYA) (**b**) obverse, (**e**) reverse, Yeast Extract Sucrose agar (YES) (**c**) obverse, (**f**) reverse, (**h**) Creatine Sucrose Agar (CREA)—strong acid production, (**g**) conidiophores and conidia. Scale: black bar = 10 µm.

Identified *P. crustosum* strains also showed good growth on MEA, CYA, and YES media. The average colony diameters were (34.10 ± 4.05) mm for MEA (34.33 ± 4.50) mm for CYA and (34.76 ± 4.90) mm for YES agar after incubation at 25 °C for 7 days. Colonies on both MEA and CYA were weakly fasciculate to crustose, dull green to grey green with corrugation and thin white edge hem. Reverse colony color on MEA was cream to beige. On CYA, copious clear or brown exudate droplets were present and reverse colony color was cream to yellow brown. Characteristic crustose colonies of grey green color with thin white edge hem and cream to yellow reverse were observed on YES medium. Conidiophores were terverticillate with rough-walled stripe, phialides cylindrical tapering to a distinct collulum. Conidia were smooth-walled, globose to subglobose. Negative Ehrlich reaction was manifested by 13 strains and good acid production was observed in 14 strains (Table 2, Figure 3).

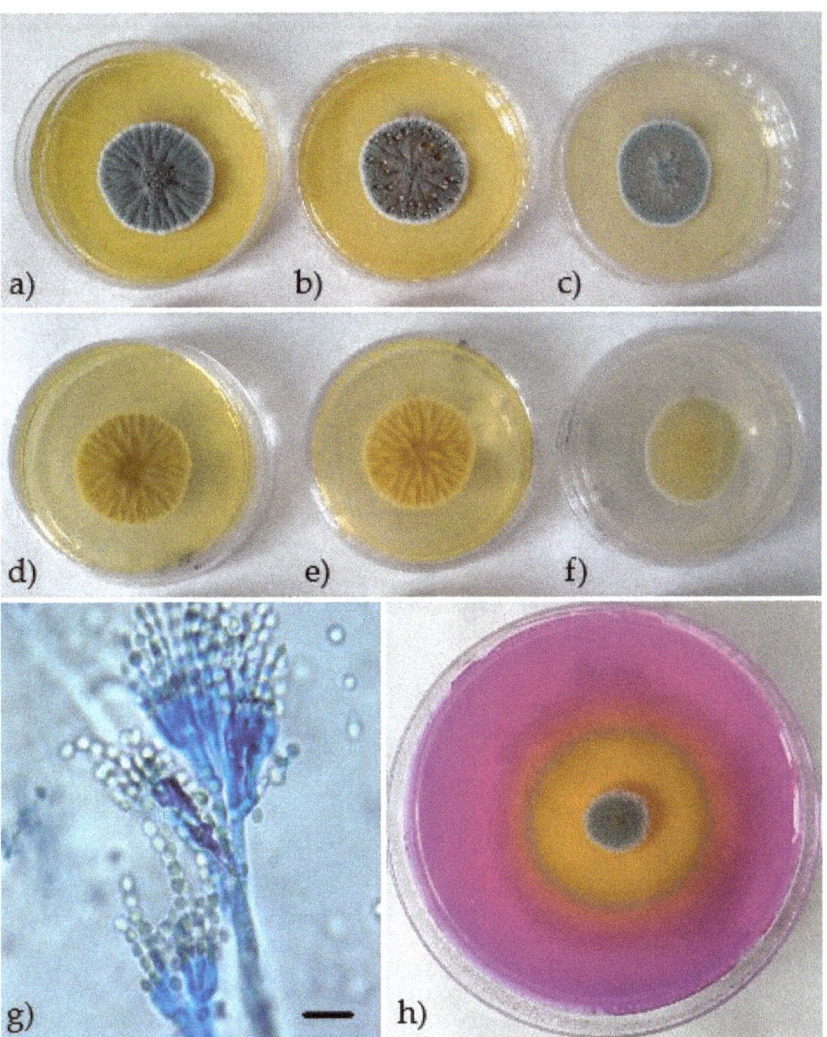

Figure 3. *Penicillium crustosum*. Seven-day-old colonies on Malt Extract Agar (MEA) (**a**) obverse, (**d**) reverse, Czapek Yeast Autolysate agar (CYA) (**b**) obverse, (**e**) reverse, Yeast Extract Sucrose agar (YES) (**c**) obverse, (**f**) reverse, (**h**) Creatine Sucrose Agar (CREA)—good acid production, (**g**) conidiophores and conidia. Scale: black bar = 10 µm.

3.2. PCR-ITS-RFLP Analysis

The ITS1 and ITS4 primers were used to amplify ITS1-5.8S-ITS2 region of rRNA, which shows low intraspecific polymorphism and high interspecific variability. PCR-ITS-RFLP was initially performed with the reference strains, where the ribosomal restriction patterns were assembled. Amplicons of size 650 bp (*P. commune* and *P. crustosum*) or 600 bp (*P. verrucosum*) were digested by seven restriction endonucleases: *Bsp1286*I, *Xma*I, *Hae*III, *Hinf*I, *Mse*I, *Sfc*I, and *Hpy188*I. Ribosomal restriction patterns of the tested strains were compared against those of particular reference strains.

Based on these results, three species within the genus *Penicillium* have been identified: *P. verrucosum*, *P. commune*, and *P. crustosum* (Table 3). Ribosomal restriction patterns of the three species after visualization by ultraviolet (UV) transillumination are presented in Figure 4.

Table 3. Species-specific identification of *Penicillium* species based on ribosomal restriction patterns.

		Fungal Species		
		P. verrucosum	*P. commune*	*P. crustosum*
Number of isolates		8	36	19
PCR amplicons (bp)		600	650	650
Restriction fragments (bp)	*Bsp1286*I	41 + 60 + 169 + 263	164 + 260	169 + 263
	*Xma*I	467 + 128	495	497 + 142
	*Hae*III	40 + 54 + 72 + 110 + 260	72 + 260	54 + 72 + 260
	*Hinf*I	112 + 180 + 298	275	300
	*Mse*I	201 + 362	101 + 353	103 + 365
	*Sfc*I	110 + 491	100 + 464	110 + 491
	*Hpy188*I	168 + 400	135 + 170	53 + 135 + 152

PCR fragments below 40 bp were not displayed.

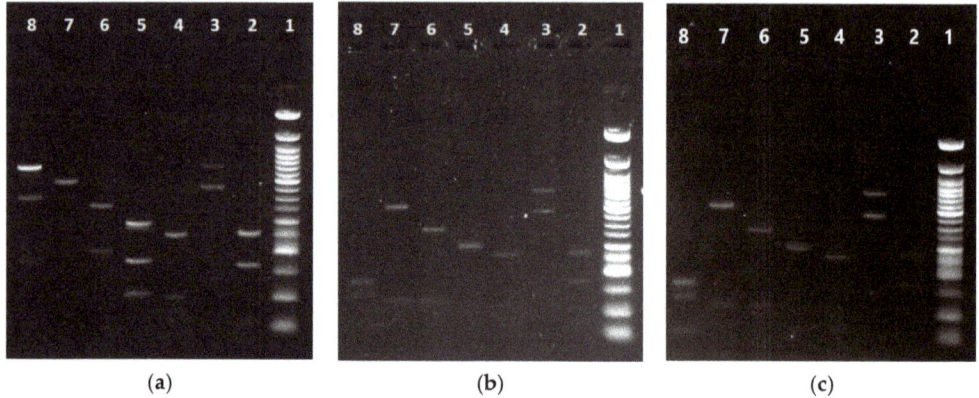

Figure 4. Restriction patterns presented by the reference strains and *Penicillium* (P.) isolates analyzed: (**a**) *P. verrucosum*. Line 1: 50 bp ladder standard; Lines 2 to 8: restriction fragments formed after digestion by endonucleases *Bsp1286*I, *Xma*I, *Hae*III, *Hinf*I, *Mse*I, *Sfc*I, and *Hpy188*I; (**b**) *P. commune*. Line 1: 50 bp ladder standard; Lines 2 to 8: restriction fragments formed after digestion by endonucleases *Bsp1286*I, *Xma*I, *Hae*III, *Hinf*I, *Mse*I, *Sfc*I, and *Hpy188*I; (**c**) *P. crustosum*. Line 1: 50 bp ladder standard; Lines 2 to 8: restriction fragments formed after digestion by endonucleases *Bsp1286*I, *Xma*I, *Hae*III, *Hinf*I, *Mse*I, *Sfc*I, and *Hpy188*I.

3.3. Identification by Conventional PCR

Penicillium strains identified with the help of PCR-ITS-RFLP were further confirmed by conventional PCR method using the primers designed on the ITS1-5.8S-ITS2 rRNA sequences. The specificity of primer pairs used in conventional PCR was tested with reference strains of seven *Penicillium* species. The expected sizes of amplicons were about 607 bp for VERF/VERR (*P. verrucosum*), 464 bp for COMF/COMR (*P. commune*), and 892 bp for CRUF/CRUR (*P. crustosum*). In the case of remaining four *Penicillium* species tested, no PCR products were displayed (Figure 5). Subsequently, *Penicillium* isolates from table eggs were tested for amplification using the same primer pairs and compared to a particular reference strain. Primers 18S-F/18S-R were used as positive amplification control in this assay (Figure 6).

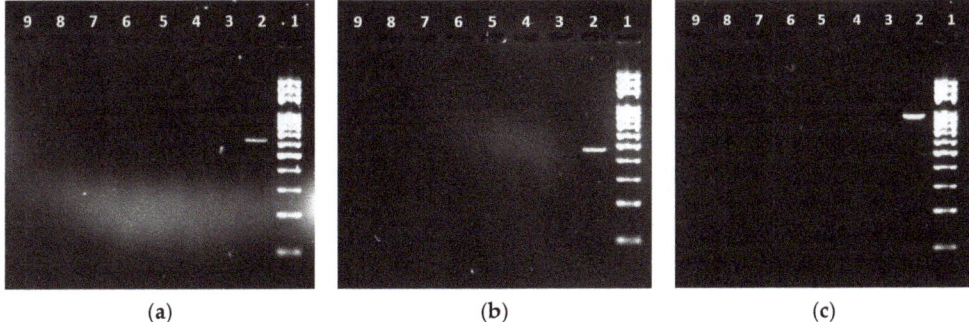

Figure 5. The specificity of primer pairs used in conventional PCR. (**a**) DNA amplicons of *Penicillium* (*P.*) reference strains using the VERF/VERR primer pair. Line 1: 100 bp ladder standard; Line 2: *P. verrucosum* (ATCC® 44407™); Line 3: negative control; Line 4 to 9: reference strains *P. commune* (CCM F-327), *P. crustosum* (CCM 8322), *P. chrysogenum* (CCM F-362), *P. brevicompactum* (CCM 8040), *P. glabrum* (CCM F-310), *P. expansum* (CCM F-576); (**b**) DNA amplicons of *Penicillium* reference strains using the COMF/COMR primer pair. Line 1: 100 bp ladder standard; Line 2: *P. commune* (CCM F-327); Line 3: negative control; Line 4 to 9: reference strains *P. verrucosum* (ATCC® 44407™); *P. crustosum* (CCM 8322), *P. chrysogenum* (CCM F-362), *P. brevicompactum* (CCM 8040), *P. glabrum* (CCM F-310), *P. expansum* (CCM F-576); (**c**) DNA amplicons of *Penicillium* reference strains using the COMF/COMR primer pair. Line 1: 100 bp ladder standard; Line 2: *P. crustosum* (CCM 8322); Line 3: negative control; Line 4 to 9: reference strains *P. verrucosum* (ATCC® 44407™); *P. commune* (CCM F-327), *P. chrysogenum* (CCM F-362), *P. brevicompactum* (CCM 8040), *P. glabrum* (CCM F-310), *P. expansum* (CCM F-576).

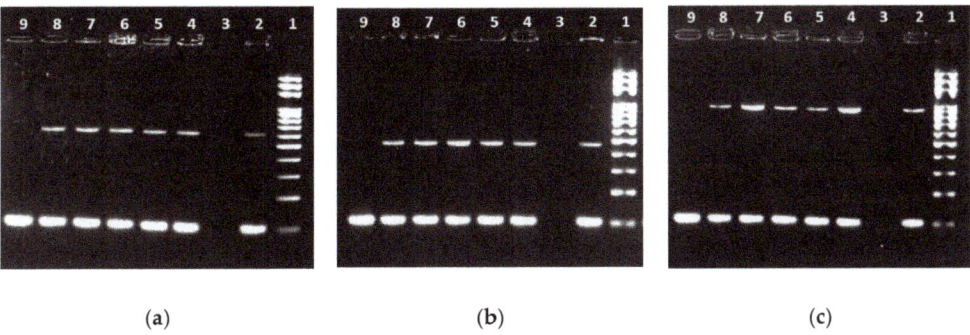

Figure 6. Electrophoretic analysis of amplicons of *Penicillium* (*P.*) isolates from table eggs by conventional PCR. (**a**) *P. verrucosum*: Line 1: 100 bp ladder standard; Line 2: *P. verrucosum* (ATCC® 44407™); Line 3: negative control; Lines 4 to 8: isolates of *P. verrucosum* (607 bp); Line 9: 18S rRNA internal control (99 bp); (**b**) *P. commune*: Line 1: 100 bp ladder standard; Line 2: *P. commune* (CCM F-327); Line 3: negative control; Lines 4 to 8: isolates of *P. commune* (464 bp); Line 9: 18S rRNA internal control (99 bp); (**c**) *P. crustosum*: Line 1: 100 bp ladder standard; Line 2: *P. crustosum* (CCM 8322); Line 3: negative comtrol; Lines 4 to 8: isolates of *P. crustosum* (892 bp); Line 9: 18S rRNA internal control (99 bp).

3.4. Comparison of Results Obtained by Three Identification Methods

Initial identification of *Penicillium* isolates was based on evaluation of both macroscopic and microscopic features. After that, more accurate identification was performed using two molecular methods.

The results of this study showed the lowest coincidence in the group of *P. verrucosum* isolates, were only eight strains, out of 12 strains identified morphologically, were confirmed by molecular methods. Among *P. commune* isolates, 42 out of 48 strains previously identified by phenotypic evaluation, were subsequently confirmed by both PCR methods. The most accurate identification was obtained for *P. crustosum*, where 21 isolates were identified morphologically and 19 isolates using both molecular methods.

4. Discussion

Accurate identification is the basis for all aspects of the diagnosis and epidemiology, whether it is pathology, medical sciences, environmental studies, or biological control. Early identification of the pathogen is crucial for the implementation of corrective actions and control measures. *Penicillium* spp. are ubiquitous microscopic filamentous fungi that have been isolated from widespread substrates. In this study, microscopic filamentous fungi of *Penicillium* spp. were isolated from the surface of chicken eggshells. Table eggs are very susceptible to fungal contamination under unsuitable storage conditions, such as increased humidity and absence of air circulation [30]. Fungal contamination of chicken eggs has been described in several studies [31–33]. Regecová et al. [26] reported the occurrence of microscopic filamentous fungi of *Penicillium* spp., *Aspergillus* spp., *Cladosporium* spp., and *Alternaria alternate* group in chicken eggs. Similar results were obtained by Rajmani et al. [34]. In the study of Neamatallah et al. [35], 38% of the eggs examined were contaminated with spores of potentially toxinogenic *Penicillium*, *Aspergillus*, and *Fusarium* species. According to Tomczyk et al. [36], fungi belonging to *Alternaria*, *Penicillium*, and *Chaetomium* spp. are the most common contaminants of the eggshell surface.

Food contamination by *Penicillium* spp. is far common in all industrial food sectors and leads to economic losses and potential risk for public health. In addition, identification of *Penicillium* species may be challenging in conventional cultivation methods. These are based on the isolation of microorganisms followed by morphological and biochemical identifications, the results of which often lead to identification problems.

For long time, *P. commune* was considered to be a fungal pathogen frequently associated with cheeses [37]. Current studies prove that *P. commune* is a cosmopolitan species with a high saprophytic ability to colonize different types of substrates [38].

P. crustosum is an important and panglobal contaminant of lipid- and protein-rich foods and feeds. This species is extremely consistent in its phenotypic properties, including morphology, physiology, and the production of secondary metabolites. However, some food isolates may differ from the others by weak growth on Creatine agar medium [14].

In this study, phenotypic identification was performed according to the identification key established by Frisvad and Samson [11]. As reported by the authors, *P. crustosum* and *P. verrucosum* do not produce cyclopiazonic acid or other alkaloids, i.e., the Ehrlich reaction should be negative. However, testing of *Penicillium* isolates in this study has also provided positive (yellow) Ehrlich reaction in some of *P. crustosum* and *P. verrucosum* strains. Similar finding were also presented by Bragulat et al. [39]. Along with strong violet reaction reported for *P. commune* strains [11,40], purple or negative reactions have also been observed in this study. As to the creatine test, weak growth of *P. verrucosum* with no acid production on CREA was expected [11]. In this study, five *P. verrucosum* isolates showed good growth on CREA and strong acid production was confirmed in four isolates. In contrary, very good growth and very good acid production on CREA were reported for both *P. crustosum* and *P. commune* strains [11]. Nevertheless, weak growth was observed in nine strains of *P. commune* and seven strains of *P. crustosum*. Weak acid production was confirmed in eleven *P. commune* isolates and seven *P. crustosum* isolates did not even produce any acid at all. Based on typical morphological and phenotypic characteristics,

Penicillium isolates were identified as *P. verrucosum*, *P. commune*, or *P. crustosum*. Some discrepancies revealed in this study could be explained by the fact that the production of secondary metabolites may not be expressed in all strains within a particular species [41]. To confirm the results of phenotypic identification, the isolates were further subjected to species-specific molecular identification.

Cultivation of molds is time-consuming, labor-intensive, non-quantitative, and susceptible to contamination and inaccuracies in classification. There is therefore a general need to design new, fast, highly specific, and reliable identification methods. In this study, two molecular methods were used for final identification of *Penicillium* species isolated from chicken eggs. As no conventional PCR assay has been available so far, three species-specific primer pairs were designed and introduced in this study to distinguish closely related species of *P. verrucosum*, *P. commune*, and *P. crustosum*. The PCR-ITS-RFLP assay was used to verify specificity and reliability of the results obtained by conventional PCR assay. Among the regions of the ribosomal cistron, the ITS region has the highest probability of successful identification for the broadest range of fungi, with the most clearly defined barcode gap between inter- and intraspecific variation [42]. The PCR-ITS-RFLP assay has high reproducibility and low cost [43,44]. Due to technical and analytical straightforwardness, it is currently considered as one of the leading fingerprinting methods [45]. In this study, different sizes of DNA restriction fragments allowed to identify all the three *Penicillium* species (*P. verrucosum*, *P. commune*, and *P. crustosum*). Diguță et al. [28] proclaimed, that the combination of nine endonucleases (*Sdu*I, *Hinf*I, *Mse*I, *Bfm*I, *Mae*II, *Cfr*9I, *Hpy188*I, and *Psp*GI) is sufficient for complete species discrimination. The identification of microscopic filamentous fungi by PCR-ITS-RFLP has been described in many studies [46–55]. The main advantage of this method is that no special equipment is required and the method can be used to identify a wide range of different microorganisms without the need to change the analytical procedure. Thus, the suitability of PCR-ITS-RFLP method for identification of microscopic filamentous fungi has also been confirmed in other studies [12,17,56–58].

Real-time PCR assays with DNA probes were also successfully used to identify *P. verrucosum* [59], *P. commune* [60], and *P. crustosum* [18]. Currently, more recent and effective methods are available for mold species identification. Among them, proteomic assays allow location-specific analysis, as well as the study of post-translational modifications (e.g., phosphorylation and glycosylation), which might impact on signal transduction in eukaryotic systems, such as fungi [61]. Metagenomic analysis can be extensive but requires more complex bioinformatic interpretation and the protocols [62].

In this study, conventional PCR method was designed and compared with both classical morphological identification assay and PCR-ITS-RFLP analysis in an attempt to reduce costs and simplify routine identification procedure of the three *Penicillium* species. Based on the results obtained it can be concluded that the traditional PCR assay is rapid and highly specific and provides an advantageous alternative to current methods significantly facilitating identification of undesirable penicillia contaminating food. As demonstrated in this study, if the results of morphological identification are not confirmed by molecular methods, the absence of key metabolic features may lead to mold species misidentification.

Both PCR methods used in this study demonstrated the ability to differentiate three *Penicillium* species at a good level. The evaluation could be probably more challenging when large numbers of samples need to be analyzed using PCR-ITS-RFLP. Considering the time and financial costs of both methods, the newly designed conventional PCR seems to be more advantageous.

Author Contributions: Conceptualization, P.J.; methodology, P.J. and I.R.; software, I.R. and S.D.; formal analysis, M.P.; investigation and data curation, S.D., P.J. and I.R.; writing—original draft preparation, S.D.; writing—review and editing, M.P.; supervision, M.P. and P.J.; project administration and funding acquisition, P.J. All authors have read and agreed to the published version of the manuscript.

Funding: This work was supported by Scientific Grant Agency of the Ministry of Education, Science, Research and Sport of the Slovak Republic and the Slovak Academy of Sciences (VEGA 1/0705/16).

Institutional Review Board Statement: Not applicable.

Informed Consent Statement: Not applicable.

Data Availability Statement: The data presented in this study are available on request from the corresponding author.

Conflicts of Interest: The authors declare no conflict of interest.

References

1. Visagie, C.M.; Houbraken, J.; Frisvad, J.C.; Hong, S.-B.; Klaassen, C.H.W.; Perrone, G.; Seifert, K.A.; Varga, J.; Yaguchi, T.; Samson, R.A. Identification and nomenclature of the genus *Penicillium*. *Stud. Mycol.* **2014**, *78*, 343–371. [CrossRef] [PubMed]
2. Samson, R.A.; Houbraken, J.; Thrane, U.; Frisvad, J.C.; Andersen, B. *Food and Indoor Fungi*, 2nd ed.; CBS Laboratory Manual Series; CBS KNAW Biodiversity Centre: Utrecht, The Netherlands, 2010; Volume 2, p. 390. ISBN 978-90-70351-82-3.
3. Storey, E.; Dangman, K.H.; Schenck, P.; DeBernardo, R.L.; Yang, C.S.; Bracker, A.; Hodgson, M.J. *Guidance for Clinicians on the Recognition and Management of Health Effects Related to Mold Exposure and Moisture Indoors*; University of Connecticut Health Center: Farmington, CT, USA, 2004; p. 17.
4. Rundberget, T.; Skaar, I.; Flåøyen, A. The presence of *Penicillium* and *Penicillium* mycotoxins in food wastes. *Int. J. Food Microbiol.* **2004**, *90*, 181–188. [CrossRef]
5. Mansour, A.F.A.; Zayed, A.F.; Basha, O.A.A. Contamination of the shell and internal content of table eggs with some pathogens during different storage periods. *Assiut Vet. Med. J.* **2015**, *61*, 8–15.
6. Commission Regulation (EC) No. 589/2008 of 23 June 2008 Laying Down Detailed Rules for Implementing Council Regulation (EC) No. 1234/2007 as Regards Marketing Standards for Eggs. Available online: https://eur-lex.europa.eu/LexUriServ/LexUriServ.do?uri=OJ:L:2008:163:0006:0023:EN:PDF (accessed on 20 October 2020).
7. Leggieri, M.C.; Pietri, A.; Battilani, P. Modelling fungal growth, mycotoxin production and release in Grana cheese. *Microorganisms* **2020**, *8*, 69. [CrossRef] [PubMed]
8. Lund, F.; Nielsen, A.B.; Skouboe, P. Distribution of *Penicillium commune* isolates in cheese dairies mapped using secondary metabolite profiles, morphotypes, RAPD and AFLP fingerprinting. *Food Microbiol.* **2003**, *20*, 20725–20734. [CrossRef]
9. Kure, C.F.; Abeln, E.C.A.; Holst-Jensen, A.; Skaar, I. Differentiation of *Penicillium commune* and *Penicillium palitans* isolates from cheese and indoor environments of cheese factories using M13 fingerprinting. *Food Microbiol.* **2002**, *19*, 151–157. [CrossRef]
10. Houbraken, J.; Visagie, C.M.; Meijer, M.; Frisvad, J.C.; Busby, P.E.; Pitt, J.I.; Seifert, K.A.; Louis-Seize, G.; Demirel, R.; Yilmaz, N.; et al. A taxonomic and phylogenetic revision of *Penicillium* section *Aspergilloides*. *Stud. Mycol.* **2014**, *78*, 373–451. [CrossRef]
11. Frisvad, J.C.; Samson, R.A. Polyphasic taxonomy of *Penicillium* subgenus *Penicillium*. A guide to identification of food and air-borne terverticillate Penicillia and their mycotoxins. *Stud. Mycol.* **2004**, *49*, 1–174.
12. Toju, H.; Tanabe, A.S.; Yamamoto, S.; Sato, H. High-coverage ITS primers for the DNA-based identification of ascomycetes and basidiomycetes in environmental samples. *PLoS ONE* **2012**, *7*, e40863. [CrossRef]
13. Koffi, Y.F.; Diguta, C.; Alloue-Boraud, M.; Ban Koffi, L.; Dje, M.; Gherghina, E.; Matei, F. PCR-ITS-RFLP identification of pineapple spoilage fungi. *Rom. Biotechnol. Lett.* **2019**, *24*, 418–424. [CrossRef]
14. Sonjak, S.; Frisvad, J.C.; Gunde-Cimerman, N. Genetic Variation among *Penicillium crustosum* isolates from arctic and other ecological niches. *Microb. Ecol.* **2007**, *54*, 298–305. [CrossRef] [PubMed]
15. Chen, R.S.; Tsay, J.G.; Huang, Y.F.; Chiou, R.Y. Polymerase chain reaction-mediated characterization of molds belonging to the *Aspergillus flavus* group and detection of *Aspergillus parasiticus* in peanut kernels by multiplex polymerase chain reaction. *J. Food Prot.* **2002**, *65*, 840–844. [CrossRef] [PubMed]
16. Apaliya, M.T.; Zhang, H.; Zheng, X.; Yang, Q.; Mahunu, G.K.; Kwaw, E. Exogenous trehalose enhanced the biocontrol efficacy of *Hanseniaspora uvarum* against grape berry rots caused by *Aspergillus tubingensis* and *Penicillium commune*. *J. Sci. Food Agric.* **2018**, *98*, 4665–4672. [CrossRef] [PubMed]
17. Dhungana, B.; Ali, S.; Byamukama, E.; Krishnan, P.; Caffe-Treml, M. Incidence of *Penicillium verrucosum* in grain samples from oat varieties commonly grown in South Dakota. *J. Food Prot.* **2018**, *81*, 898–902. [CrossRef]
18. Gonda, M.; Rufo, C.; Cecchetto, G.; Vero, S. Evaluation of different hurdles on *Penicillium crustosum* growth in sponge cakes by means of a specific real time PCR. *J. Food Sci. Technol.* **2019**, *56*, 2195–2204. [CrossRef]
19. Al-Anati, L.; Petzinger, E. Immunotoxic activity of ochratoxin A. *J. Vet. Pharmacol. Ther.* **2006**, *29*, 79–90. [CrossRef]
20. Frisvad, J.C.; Smedsgaard, J.; Larsen, T.O.; Samson, R.A. Mycotoxins, drugs and other extrolites produced by species in *Penicillium* subgenus *Penicillium*. *Stud. Mycol.* **2004**, *49*, 201–241.
21. Moldes-Anaya, A.; Rundberget, T.; Fæste, C.K.; Eriksen, G.S.; Bernhoft, A. Neurotoxicity of *Penicillium crustosum* secondary metabolites: Tremorgenic activity of orally administered penitrem A and thomitrem A and E in mice. *Toxicon* **2012**, *60*, 1428–1435. [CrossRef]
22. Vinokurova, N.G.; Ozerskaya, S.M.; Baskunov, B.P.; Arinbasarov, M.U. The *Penicillium commune* Thom and *Penicillium clavigerum* Demelius fungi—Fumigaclavines A and B producers. *Mikrobiologiia* **2003**, *72*, 180–182. [CrossRef]

23. Wagener, R.E.; Davis, N.D.; Diener, U.L. Penitrem A and Roquefortine Production by *Penicillium commune*. *Appl. Environ. Microbiol.* **1980**, *39*, 882–887. [CrossRef]
24. STN ISO 21527-1. *Microbiology of Food and Animal Feeding Stuffs. Horizontal Method for the Enumeration of Yeasts and Molds. Part 1: Colony Count Technique in Products with Water Activity Greater than 0.95*; ISO 21527-1:2008; Slovak Standards Institute: Bratislava, Slovak Republic, 2010.
25. STN ISO 21527-2. *Microbiology of Food and Animal Feeding Stuffs. Horizontal Method for the Enumeration of Yeasts and Molds. Part 2: Colony Count Technique in Products with Water Activity less than or Equal to 0.95*; ISO 21527-2:2008; Slovak Standards Institute: Bratislava, Slovak Republic, 2010.
26. Regecová, I.; Pipová, M.; Jevinová, P.; Demjanová, S.; Semjon, B. Quality and mycobiota composition of stored eggs. *Ital. J. Food Sci.* **2020**, *32*, 540–561. [CrossRef]
27. White, T.J.; Bruns, T.D.; Lee, S.B.; Taylor, J.W. Amplification and direct sequencing of fungal ribosomal RNA genes for phylogenetics. In *PCR Protocols: A Guide to Methods and Applications*; Innis, M.A., Gelfand, D.H., Sninsky, J.J., White, T.J., Eds.; Academic Press: New York, NY, USA, 1990; pp. 315–322. ISBN -978-0-12372180-8. [CrossRef]
28. Diguță, C.F.; Vincent, B.; Guilloux-Benatier, M.; Alexandre, H.; Rousseaux, S. PCR ITS-RFLP: A useful method for identifying filamentous fungi isolates on grapes. *Food Microbiol.* **2011**, *28*, 1145–1154. [CrossRef] [PubMed]
29. López-Andreo, M.; Lugo, L.; Garrido-Pertierra, A.; Prieto, M.I.; Puyet, A. Identification and quantitation of species in complex DNA mixtures by real-time polymerase chain reaction. *Anal. Biochem.* **2005**, *339*, 73–82. [CrossRef] [PubMed]
30. Al-Obaidi, F.A.; Al-Shadeedi, S.M.J.; Al-Dalawi, R.H. Quality, chemical and microbial characteristics of table eggs at retail stores in Baghdad. *Inter. J. Poultry. Sci.* **2011**, *10*, 381–385. [CrossRef]
31. Perez-Nadales, E.; Nogueira, M.D.; Baldwin, C.; Castanheira, S.E.; Ghalid, M.; Grund, E.; Lengeler, K.; Marchegiani, E.; Mehrotra, P.V.; Moretti, M.; et al. Fungal model systems and the elucidation of pathogenicity determinants. *Fungal Genet. Biol.* **2014**, *70*, 42–67. [CrossRef] [PubMed]
32. Hassan, Z.U.; Ahmad, S. Transfer of mycotoxin residues in hen's egg, their interaction and mechanism. In *Handbook of Eggs in Human Function. Human Health Handbooks*; Watson, R.R., De Meester, F., Eds.; Wageningen Academic Publishers: Wageningen, The Netherlands, 2015; Volume 9, pp. 365–386. ISBN 978-90-8686-254-2. [CrossRef]
33. Rodríguez, A.; Rodríguez, M.; Anreade, M.J.; Córdoba, J.J. Detection of filamentous fungi in foods. *Curr. Opin. Food. Sci.* **2015**, *5*, 36–42. [CrossRef]
34. Rajmani, R.S.; Singh, A.P.; Singh, P.K.; Doley, J.; Verma, S.P. Fungal contamination in eggs. *J. Vet. Pub. Health* **2011**, *9*, 59–61. [CrossRef]
35. Neamatallah, A.A.; El-Leboudy, A.; Amer, A.A.; El-Shenawy, N.M. Biosafety against fungal contamination of hen's eggs and mycotoxins producing species. *JKAU Met. Environ. Arid Land Agric. Sci.* **2009**, *20*, 63–73. [CrossRef]
36. Tomczyk, Ł.; Stępień, Ł.; Urbaniak, M.; Szablewski, T.; Cegielska-Radziejewska, R.; Stuper-Szablewska, K. Characterisation of the mycobiota on the shell surface of table eggs acquired from different egg-laying hen breeding systems. *Toxins* **2018**, *10*, 293. [CrossRef]
37. Ramos-Pereiraa, J.; Marezeb, J.; Patrinoua, E.; Santosa, J.A.; Lopez-Diaza, T.-M. Polyphasic identification of *Penicillium* spp. isolated from Spanish semi-hard ripened cheeses. *Food Microbiol.* **2019**, *84*, 103253:1–103253:8. [CrossRef]
38. Rodríguez, R.D.; Heredia, G.; Siles, J.A.; Jurado, M.; Saparrat, M.C.N.; García-Romera, I.; Sampedro, I. Enhancing laccase production by white-rot fungus *Funalia floccosa* LPSC 232 in co-culture with *Penicillium commune* GHAIE86. *Folia Microbiol.* **2019**, *64*, 91–99. [CrossRef] [PubMed]
39. Bragulat, M.R.; Martínez, E.; Castellá, G.; Cabañes, F.J. Ochratoxin A and citrinin producing species of the genus *Penicillium* from feedstuffs. *Int. J. Food Microbiol.* **2008**, *126*, 43–48. [CrossRef] [PubMed]
40. Zhelifonova, V.P.; Antipova, T.V.; Kozlovskii, A.G. Effect of potassium sorbate, sodium benzoate, and sodium nitrite on biosynthesis of cyclopiazonic and mycophenolic acids and citrinin by fungi of the *Penicillium* genus. *Appl. Biochem. Microbiol.* **2017**, *53*, 711–714. [CrossRef]
41. Pitt, J.I.; Hocking, A.D. *Fungi and Food Spoilage*, 3rd ed.; Springer Science & Business Media: New York, NY, USA, 2009; ISBN 978-0-387-92207-2. [CrossRef]
42. Schoch, C.L.; Seifert, K.A.; Huhndorf, S.; Robert, V.; Spouge, J.L.; Levesque, C.A.; Chen, W. Fungal Barcoding Consortium. Nuclear ribosomal internal transcribed spacer (ITS) region as a universal DNA barcode marker for Fungi. *PNAS* **2012**, *109*, 6241–6246. [CrossRef] [PubMed]
43. Thies, J.E. Soil microbial community analysis using terminal restriction fragment length polymorphisms. *SSSA J.* **2007**, *71*, 579–591. [CrossRef]
44. Cao, Y.; Van De Werfhorst, L.C.; Dubinsky, E.A.; Badgley, B.D.; Sadowsky, M.J.; Andersen, G.L.; Griffith, J.F.; Holden, P.A. Evaluation of molecular community analysis methods for discerning fecal sources and human waste. *Water Res.* **2013**, *47*, 6862–6872. [CrossRef]
45. Schütte, U.M.E.; Abdo, Z.; Bent, S.J.; Shyu, C.; Williams, C.J.; Pierson, J.D.; Forney, L.J. Advances in the use of terminal restriction fragment length polymorphism (T-RFLP) analysis of 16S rRNA genes to characterize microbial communities. *Appl. Microbiol. Biotechnol.* **2008**, *80*, 365–380. [CrossRef] [PubMed]
46. Khalil, M.I. Identification of *Cladosporium* sp. Fungi by in- silico RFLP-PCR. *Baghdad Sci. J.* **2020**, *17*, 220–226. [CrossRef]

47. Leite, L.N.; Lelis, F.J.N.; de Sousa Xavier, M.A.; dos Santos, J.; Cardoso, L.; Barbosa, F.S.; dos Santos, R.F.; Dias, S.A.M.; de Oliveira Xavier, A.R.E. Molecular identification and characterization of filamentous fungi and yeasts isolated in a pharmaceutical industry environment. *J. Appl. Pharm. Sci.* **2020**, *10*, 27–36. [CrossRef]
48. Szekely, J.; Chelae, S.; Ingviya, N.; Rukchang, W.; Auepemkiate, S.; Aiempanakit, K. Universal Multiplex Polymerase Chain Reaction-Restriction Fragment Length Polymorphism (UMPCR-RFLP) for rapid detection and species identification of fungal and mycobacterial pathogens. *Walailak J. Sci. Tech.* **2020**, *17*, 1113–1125. [CrossRef]
49. Kordalewska, M.; Kalita, J.; Bakuła, Z.; Brillowska-Dąbrowska, A.; Jagielski, T. PCR-RFLP assays for species-specific identification of fungi belonging to *Scopulariopsis* and related genera. *Med. Mycol.* **2019**, *57*, 643–648. [CrossRef] [PubMed]
50. Worasilchai, N.; Chaumpluk, P.; Chakrabarti, A.; Chindamporn, A. Differential diagnosis for pythiosis using thermophilic helicase DNA amplification and restriction fragment length polymorphism (tHDA-RFLP). *Med. Mycol.* **2018**, *56*, 216–224. [CrossRef] [PubMed]
51. Atoui, A.; El Khoury, A. PCR-RFLP for *Aspergillus* species. In *Mycotoxigenic Fungi. Methods in Molecular Biology*; Moretti, A., Susca, A., Eds.; Humana Press: New York, NY, USA, 2017; Volume 1542, ISBN 978-1-4939-6707-0. [CrossRef]
52. Kim, J.S.; Kang, N.J.; Kwak, Y.S.; Lee, C. Investigation of Genetic Diversity of *Fusarium oxysporum* f. sp. *fragariae* using PCR-RFLP. *Plant. Pathol. J.* **2017**, *33*, 140–147. [CrossRef] [PubMed]
53. Rousseaux, S.; Guilloux-Bénatier, M. PCR ITS-RFLP for *Penicillium* species and other genera. In *Mycotoxigenic Fungi. Methods in Molecular Biology*; Moretti, A., Susca, A., Eds.; Humana Press: New York, NY, USA, 2017; Volume 1542, ISBN 978-1-4939-6707-0. [CrossRef]
54. Srivastava, S.; Gupta, P.S.; Lal, S.; Sinha, O.K. Rapid identification of endophytic fungi of sugarcan (saccharum spp. hybrid) using PCR-RFLP of rDNA. *J. Environ. Biol.* **2017**, *38*, 21–26. [CrossRef]
55. Grudzinska-Sterno, M.; Yuen, J.; Stenlid, J.; Djurle, A. Fungal communities in organically grown winter wheat affected by plant organ and development stage. *Eur. J. Plant. Pathol.* **2016**, *146*, 401–417. [CrossRef]
56. Diguță, C.F.; Toma, R.C.; Cornea, C.P.; Matei, F. Molecular detection of black *Aspergillus* and *Penicillium* species from Dealu Mare vineyard. *Sci. Pap. Ser. B Hortic.* **2018**, *62*, 305–310.
57. De Sousa, D.R.T.; da Silva Santos, C.S.; Wanke, B.; da Silva, R.M., Jr.; dos Santos, M.C.; Cruz, K.S.; Monte, R.L.; Nocker, A.; de Souza, J.V.B. PCR-RFLP as a useful tool for diagnosis of invasive mycoses in a healthcare facility in the North of Brazil. *Electron. J. Biotechnol.* **2015**, *18*, 231–235. [CrossRef]
58. Ziaee, A.; Zia, M.; Bayat, M.; Hashemi, J. Molecular Identification of *Mucor* and *Lichtheimia* species in pure cultures of *Zygomycetes*. *Jundishapur J. Microbiol.* **2016**, *9*, e35237:1–e35237:8. [CrossRef]
59. Vegi, A.; Wolf-Hall, C.E. Multiplex real-time PCR method for detection and quantification of mycotoxigenic fungi belonging to three different genera. *J. Food Sci.* **2013**, *78*, M70–M76. [CrossRef]
60. Rodríguez, A.; Luque, M.I.; Andrade, M.J.; Rodríguez, M.; Asensio, M.A.; Córdoba, J.J. Development of real-time PCR methods to quantify patulin-producing molds in food products. *Food Microbiol.* **2011**, *28*, 1190–1199. [CrossRef]
61. Pandey, A.; Mann, M. Proteomics to study genes and genomes. *Nature* **2000**, *405*, 837–846. [CrossRef] [PubMed]
62. Balint, M.; Bahram, M.; Murat Eren, A.; Faust, K.; Fuhrman, J.A.; Orn Lindahl, B.; O'Hara, R.B.; Opik, M.; Sogin, M.L.; Unterseher, M.; et al. Millions of reads, thousands of taxa: Microbial community structure and associations analyzed via marker genes FEMS microbiology reviews advance access. *FEMS Microbiol. Rev.* **2016**, *40*, 686–700. [CrossRef] [PubMed]

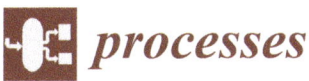

Article

Effect of *Cladosporium cladosporioides* on the Composition of Mycoflora and the Quality Parameters of Table Eggs during Storage

Pavlina Jevinová, Monika Pipová *, Ivana Regecová, Soňa Demjanová, Boris Semjon, Slavomír Marcinčák, Jozef Nagy and Ivona Kožárová

Department of Food Hygiene, Technology and Safety, University of Veterinary Medicine and Pharmacy, Komenského 73, 041 81 Košice, Slovakia; pavlina.jevinova@uvlf.sk (P.J.); ivana.regecova@uvlf.sk (I.R.); sona.demjanova@student.uvlf.sk (S.D.); boris.semjon@uvlf.sk (B.S.); slavomir.marcincak@uvlf.sk (S.M.); jozef.nagy@uvlf.sk (J.N.); ivona.kozarova@uvlf.sk (I.K.)
* Correspondence: monika.pipova@uvlf.sk; Tel.: +421-915984562

Abstract: The eggshells of 120 experimental one-day-old table eggs were contaminated with the spore suspension of *Cladosporium cladosporioides*, divided into three groups (A–C) and stored at three different temperatures (3 °C, 11 °C and 20 °C) for 28 days. Visible growth of molds on/in experimental eggs was not observed within the entire storage period. No significant differences in the numbers of molds were found between particular groups of eggs. However, the composition of egg mycoflora was greatly influenced by storage conditions. Three mold genera were identified using the PCR method. The highest mold numbers were determined on Day 14 (Groups A and C) and Day 21 (Group B) when the maximum relative humidity and dew point temperature were recorded. On the same days, the dominance of *Penicillium* spp. and the minimum eggshell firmness were observed. Noticeable changes in egg quality were observed in eggs stored at 20 °C, and most of these eggs were downgraded at the end of storage period. The growth ability differed significantly among three mold genera. *Penicillium* spp. and *Fusarium* spp. showed better growth intensity at increased values (0.91–0.94) of water activity (a_w) indicating a possible risk associated with the occurrence of mycotoxins in the egg contents.

Keywords: egg quality; mold; *Cladosporium*; *Penicillium*; *Fusarium*

1. Introduction

Cladosporium (*C.*) spp. belong to the most common molds in indoor and outdoor air, as well as in materials such as soil, plants, textiles, plastics and foodstuffs [1–6]. Small, dry and heavily pigmented conidia provide fungus with very effective protection against ultraviolet radiation and enable a long-term persistence in environments including various substrates [7]. According to the most recent information, *Cladosporium* genus includes 218 species classified into three species complexes—*C. herbarum*, *C. sphaerospermum* and *C. cladosporioides* [4,7–9]. Both *C. sphaerospermum* and *C. cladosporioides* have already been isolated from foodstuffs, indoor air and materials from households [1,7]. The presence of *C. cladosporioides* was reported in fresh vegetables, wheat, flour, barley, rice, dried fish, cheeses, sea salt, as well as in table eggs [10–12].

The risk of egg contamination is related to the penetration of microorganisms from the outside environment through the natural protective egg barriers into the egg contents [13]. With the exception of endogenous contamination, the contents of freshly laid eggs usually do not show any presence of microorganisms. The eggshell becomes contaminated with faeces in the cloaca at the moment of oviposition. Further contamination of the shell occurs immediately after laying and results from direct contact with contaminated surfaces, floor litter or nesting materials [14]. As soon as the eggshell has been exposed to the environment, it becomes heavily contaminated with various microorganisms, including the spores of molds that are therefore permanently present on the eggshell surface. Spore numbers depend on the level of contamination on egg farms and establishments for further handling and grading of eggs. Salem et al. [15] reported significantly higher numbers of spores on the surface of visibly contaminated eggshells (5.6 log CFU/g) compared with those that were uncontaminated (4.4 log CFU/g). Although the spectrum of mold species varies considerably, the most frequent mold genera found on the shell surface include *Aspergillus* spp., *Penicillium* spp., *Cladosporium* spp., *Rhizopus* spp. and *Mucor* spp. [16–18].

Generally, foods of animal origin (including table eggs) have a limited shelf life at low storage temperatures. When stored under suitable conditions (i.e., at low temperature and high relative humidity), germination of spores and growth of contaminating mycoflora are observed. Hyphae of molds are able to penetrate through the shell pores into the egg contents. This process is accompanied by the destruction of both shell membranes, thus enabling further bacterial growth. At the final stage of mold decomposition, coagulation or gelatinization of the egg albumen is observed and an unpleasant 'moldy' smell is developed, which persists even after heat processing. In such a way, table eggs become devalued and inappropriate for human consumption [19].

Due to its psychrophilic nature and growth ability at low temperatures (up to $-5\,°C$), *C. cladosporioides* is capable of causing undesirable changes in table eggs during storage. This fungal species is reported to grow at a temperature of $25\,°C$ and water activity (a_w) below 0.86 [20,21].

The aim of this study was to reveal the effect of storage conditions on the growth of molds and the related changes in the quality of table eggs previously contaminated with spores of *C. cladosporioides* during the shelf-life period.

2. Materials and Methods

2.1. Materials

The experiment was performed with 120 one-day-old table eggs. Eggshells were contaminated by the short immersion of experimental eggs into the spore suspension of *C. cladosporioides* CCM F-348 (Czech Collection of Microorganisms, Brno, Czech Republic) standardized to the density of a McFarland 0.8 turbidity standard, approximately corresponding to 6.4 log CFU/mL. After drying the shells in air, table eggs were divided into three groups (40 eggs per group), placed into cardboard boxes and stored under different conditions commonly used for the storage of eggs in households.

Group A eggs were stored in the refrigerator with forced-air convection (Liebherr, Ochsenhausen, Germany) at an average temperature of $11\,°C$. Group B eggs were kept in the refrigerator without forced-air convection (AEG, Berlin, Germany) at $3\,°C$, and Group C eggs were stored at laboratory temperature ($20\,°C$). Storage temperature, relative air humidity and dew point temperature were monitored permanently within the entire storage period using the Temperature Humidity Transmitter TFA 30.3180.IT TTH (ELSO Philips Service s.r.o., Trenčín, Slovakia). Shell surface, egg albumen and egg yolk were sampled on Days 7, 14, 21 and 28 of the experiment for enumeration of molds and evaluation of selected qualitative parameters. Shell firmness was determined with the help of the Egg Force Reader (Orka Food Technology Ltd., Herzliya, Israel), and the Egg Analyzer™ (Orka Food Technology Ltd., Herzliya, Israel) was used for automatic measurements of the egg weight, the yolk color, automatic calculation of Haugh units and assessment egg quality grades.

2.2. Enumeration of Molds

Molds were removed from the eggshell surface as described by Cupáková et al. [22]. Five eggs from each experimental group were tested every week. Each individual egg was transferred aseptically into a sterile plastic bag, and sterile peptone water (0.1%) in a volume of 100 mL had been added. The sample was then shaken for 15 min using the Orbi-ShakerTMJR (BioTech s.r.o., Bratislava, Slovakia).

Shell surface was decontaminated with alcohol and then cut with the help of a sterile scalpel. Egg yolk and egg albumen were captured separately into sterile containers. A test sample of the egg albumen/yolk in the amount of 10 g was homogenized with 90 mL of sterile peptone water (0.1%) for 2.5 min using the peristaltic BagMixer (Interscience, Nom la Brétèche, France). Decimal dilutions were prepared in accordance with STN EN ISO 6887-1 [23]. A volume of 0.1 mL of each appropriate decimal dilution was spread on the surface of Dichloran Rose Bengal Chloramphenicol agar medium (DRBC, Oxoid, Hampshire, UK). Colonies of molds were enumerated after incubation of the inoculated plates at 25 °C for 5 days [24].

2.3. Identification of Mold Genera

Colonies of molds were first identified visually on the surface of Czapek Yeast Extract Agar (CYEA), Yeast Extract Sucrose agar medium (YES), Sabouraud Dextrose Agar (SDA) and Potato Dextrose Agar (PDA, Oxoid, Hampshire, UK) within a 7-day incubation period. The following parameters were evaluated: growth rate; size, margin, morphology and radial ornamentation of the colony; color, structure and height of the aerial mycelium; and production of soluble pigments and exudates. Microscopic patterns of mold isolates were observed on slides using the lactophenol cotton blue staining procedure. The typical structure of hyphae, conidial chains, branching patterns, and sexual and asexual reproduction structures were identified using light microscopy [8,25,26].

2.4. Genus Confirmation with the Help of PCR Method

Due to the typical cell wall structure, both pre-isolation and isolation steps were used to obtain DNA from mold isolates. Mycelium in a quantity of 10–50 mg was removed from the surface of CYEA using a sterile scalpel and transferred into an Eppendorf tube with 0.2 mL of sterile zircon and glass beads (1:1 ratio). Proteinase K (Macherey-Nagel GmbH & Co., Dueren, Germany) in a volume of 10 µL was added to the sample, and the Eppendorf was incubated at 37 °C for 30 min. After incubation, 800 µL of the lysing solution FG1 (OMEGA Bio-tek, Inc., Norcross, GA, USA) was added to the sample, and the Eppendorf was incubated for another 10 min at 65 °C in ultrasound waves of 500 Hz. Subsequently, isolation of DNA was performed according to the instructions of commercially available E.Z.N.A.® Fungal DNA Mini Kit (OMEGA Bio-tek, Inc., Norcross, GA, USA). The purity and concentration of DNA obtained was checked with the help of BioSpec Nanometer Spectrophotometer (Shimadzu, Kjóto, Japan).

The forward primer Pen 1–F (5′-AAATATAAATTATTTAAAACTTTC-3′) and the reverse primer Pen 2–R (5′-CTGGATAAAAATTTGGGTTG-3′) were designed based on the Internal Transcribed Spacer (ITS) region and 5.8S rRNA sequences from *Penicillium* spp. available in the GenBank-EMBL [27]. Another two primers were designed to amplify fragments within the ITS regions of *Fusarium* spp. and then synthesized commercially by Amplia s.r.o. (Bratislava, Slovakia). The initial tests for specificity have revealed that the primer pair ITS-Fu-f (5′-CAACTC CCAAACCCCTGTGA-3′) and ITS-Fu-r (5′-GCGACGATTACCAGTAACGA-3′) is highly specific for *Fusarium* genus [28].

Mitochondrial small subunit rRNA of *Cladosporium* spp. was amplified using the universal fungal mitochondrial primers MS1 (5′-CAGCAGTCAAGAATATTAGTCAATG-3′) and MS2 (5′-GCGGATTATCGAATTAAATAAC-3′). Two specific primers, Clado-PF (5′-TACTCCAATGGTTCTAATATTTTCCTCTC-3′) and Clado-PR (5′-GGGTACCTAGACAGTA TTTCTAGCCT-3′), were designed for multiplex PCR assay and synthesized by Amplia s.r.o. (Bratislava, Slovakia). The expected amplicon size for the primer pair Clado-PF/R was 87 bp [29].

The amplification was performed in the Thermal Cycler TC-512 (Techne, Stadfforshire, UK) using the PCR mixture containing 1–10 µL of template DNA, 0.5 µL of each primer (concentration 10 pmol.µL^{-1}) and 4.0 µL of HOT Firepol® Blend Master Mix (Solis BioDyne, Tartu, Estonia) in a volume of 20 µL. The same amplification conditions were used for each of the primer sets: an initial denaturation of 12 min at 95 °C was necessary for activating

HOT Firepol polymerase, followed by 30 cycles of denaturation of 20 s at 95 °C, annealing of 60 s at different temperatures for each particular primer pair (46 °C for Pen1/Pen2; 55 °C for ITS-Fu-f/ITS-Fu-r; 51 °C for MS1/MS2 and Clado-PF/Clado-PR), elongation of 2 min at 72 °C, and final extension of 10 min at 72 °C. The final amplification temperature was 6 °C.

To determine the minimum amount of fungal DNA detectable by the established PCR assays, variable quantities of mold genomic DNA ranging from 10 to 100 ng were used as the DNA template. All the PCR products were size fractionated in agarose gels (1.5%), stained with the GelRed™Nucleic Acid gel stain (Biotium, Inc., Fremont, CA, USA) and visualized by the UV transilluminator Mini Bis Pro® (DNR Bio-Imaging Systems Ltd., Neve Yamin, Izrael). Sequences obtained from the studied mold isolates were submitted to the GenBank-EMBL database and searched for homology using the Basic Local Alignment Search Tool (BLAST) program (NCBI software package).

Data generated in this study are included in this article. Sequence data that confirm mold genera identified in this study can be found in the GenBank under the following accession numbers: FJ362555.1, FN386269.1 and MH517445.1.

2.5. Characteristics of Growth and Interactions of Selected Mold Species

Spore germination and growth intensity of C. cladosporioides CCM F-348, C. herbarum, P. chrysogenum CCM F-362, P. crustosum CCM F-8322, P. griseofulvum CCM F-8006, P. glabrum CCM F-310 and F. graminearum CCM F-683 obtained from the Czech Collection of Microorganisms (CCM, Brno, Czech Republic) were tested on both DRBC and SDA. Culture media were prepared in accordance with the manufacturer's instructions. As soon as they became solid, water activity at 25 °C was measured using the LabMASTER-a_w (Novasina, Farmingdale, NY, USA). Fungal spore suspensions were adjusted to a McFarland 0.8 turbidity standard corresponding with a density of 6.4 log CFU/mL. After that, 10 µL aliquots of individual spore suspensions were applied to 6 mm sterile disks (BBL™, Los Angeles, CA, USA) placed on the surface of both DRBC and SDA agar plates. To test the spore germination and growth intensity, a single disk with spore suspension was placed to the center of a small size Petri dish (Ø 60 mm). To study fungal interactions, one disk was placed at the center of a medium size Petri dish (Ø 90 mm) and another four disks surrounded the central one at a distance of 1 cm. Fungal spore suspension was applied on the disks in various combinations in order to observe mutual interactions. After incubation of the inoculated plates at 25 °C for 120 h, both the spore germination and growth of hyphae were evaluated using the optical microscope (Lupa Hama, Monheim, Germany) at 10× magnification. As soon as visible colonies appeared on the culture media, the diameters were measured in 24-h intervals. The evaluation of mutual antifungal activity between C. cladosporioides, Penicillium and Fusarium species was based on the overall ability of a particular fungal strain to inhibit the radial growth of competitive mold genera.

2.6. Statistical Analysis

Pearson's correlation coefficients, two-way analysis of variance (ANOVA) and Tukey test for multiple comparison of means with a confidence interval set at 95% were conducted with R—statistics software. The effect of different storage conditions and the effect of the storage period were set as the main factors. Multiple factor analysis (MFA) was conducted in R—statistics software [30] with the "FactoMineR" [31] and "Factoextra" package [32] according to Semjon et al. [33].

3. Results

3.1. Effect of Storage Conditions on the Growth of C. cladosporioides and Competetive Fungal Species

In order to maintain stable storage conditions, three parameters (air temperature, relative humidity and dew point temperature) were permanently monitored during the entire storage period in this study. As seen in Table 1, storage parameters were significantly different for each of three experimental groups of table eggs ($p < 0.001$). During storage, significant differences have been observed among storage temperatures in Group C ($p < 0.01$) as well as among the values of both relative humidity and dew point temperature in Group B ($p < 0.05$). However, the highest values of both the relative humidity and the dew point temperature were recorded on Day 14 (Groups A and C) and Day 21 (Group B).

Results of the quantitative mycological examination are shown in Table 2. No significant effect of storage conditions on the numbers of molds on the shell surface or in the egg contents was confirmed in Groups A and B. Conversely, storage period significantly influenced the number of molds on the shell surface of Group C eggs ($p < 0.01$). As seen in Table 2, the average mold numbers on/in the eggs remained practically unchanged across the entire storage period and did not show any statistical significance.

Table 1. Storage conditions for three experimental groups of table eggs (mean ± SD).

Parameter	Group	Storage Period [Days]				ANOVA [p Values]	
		7	14	21	28	Impact of Storage Conditions	Impact of Storage Period
Temperature [°C]	A	11.50 ± 0.30 ^{a2}	11.44 ± 0.14 ^{a2}	11.34 ± 0.15 ^{a2}	11.46 ± 0.27 ^{a2}	$p < 0.001$	$p > 0.05$
	B	2.27 ± 0.55 ^{a3}	3.19 ± 0.90 ^{a3}	4.13 ± 1.55 ^{a3}	3.72 ± 0.77 ^{a3}		
	C	20.19 ± 0.78 ^{b1}	22.09 ± 0.13 ^{a1}	20.00 ± 0.86 ^{b1}	20.12 ± 0.36 ^{b1}		
Relative humidity [%]	A	78.75 ± 4.38 ^{a1}	80.98 ± 1.41 ^{a1}	80.02 ± 2.53 ^{a1}	76.25 ± 1.09 ^{a1}	$p < 0.001$	$p > 0.05$
	B	54.00 ± 5.00 ^{b2}	54.30 ± 4.39 ^{ab2}	64.00 ± 2.62 ^{a1}	58.74 ± 2.04 ^{ab2}		
	C	45.44 ± 2.87 ^{a2}	45.47 ± 1.49 ^{a3}	41.72 ± 11.99 ^{a2}	40.75 ± 3.42 ^{a3}		
Dew point [°C]	A	7.93 ± 0.54 ^{a1}	8.28 ± 0.19 ^{a1}	8.00 ± 0.37 ^{a1}	7.38 ± 0.31 ^{a1}	$p < 0.001$	$p > 0.05$
	B	−6.43 ± 0.32 ^{b2}	−4.83 ± 1.27 ^{ab2}	−2.07 ± 1.63 ^{a2}	−3.68 ± 1.20 ^{ab2}		
	C	8.02 ± 1.59 ^{a1}	9.76 ± 0.40 ^{a1}	6.26 ± 3.19 ^{a1}	6.36 ± 1.56 ^{a1}		

Different superscripts in the same row ($^{a, b}$) or column ($^{1-3}$) indicate that mean values differ significantly (Tukey's test, $p < 0.05$).

Table 2. Numbers of molds in experimental groups of table eggs during the storage period (mean ± SD).

Parameter	Group	Storage Period [Days]				ANOVA [p Values]	
		7	14	21	28	Impact of Storage Conditions	Impact of Storage Period
Eggshell [log CFU/egg]	A	4.37 ± 0.31 ^{a}	4.61 ± 0.12 ^{a}	4.10 ± 0.17 ^{a}	4.23 ± 0.72 ^{a}	$p < 0.001$	$p > 0.05$
	B	4.29 ± 0.03 ^{a}	4.67 ± 0.06 ^{a}	4.75 ± 0.43 ^{a}	4.28 ± 0.10 ^{a}		
	C	4.29 ± 0.17 ^{ab}	4.78 ± 0.27 ^{a}	4.42 ± 0.15 ^{ab}	3.98 ± 0.32 ^{b}		
Egg albumen [log CFU/g]	A	0.00 ± 0.00 ^{a}	2.00 ± 1.73 ^{a}	0.67 ± 1.15 ^{a}	0.87 ± 1.50 ^{a}	$p < 0.001$	$p > 0.05$
	B	0.00 ± 0.00 ^{a}	0.67 ± 1.15 ^{a}	2.19 ± 1.90 ^{a}	0.67 ± 1.15 ^{a}		
	C	0.00 ± 0.00 ^{a}	1.77 ± 1.53 ^{a}	0.67 ± 1.15 ^{a}	0.00 ± 0.00 ^{a}		
Egg yolk [log CFU/g]	A	0.00 ± 0.00 ^{a}	1.97 ± 1.71 ^{a}	0.00 ± 0.00 ^{a}	0.00 ± 0.00 ^{a}	$p < 0.001$	$p > 0.05$
	B	0.00 ± 0.00 ^{a}	0.67 ± 1.15 ^{a}	2.18 ± 1.89 ^{a}	0.67 ± 1.15 ^{a}		
	C	0.00 ± 0.00 ^{a}	1.91 ± 1.66 ^{a}	0.00 ± 0.00 ^{a}	0.67 ± 1.15 ^{a}		

Different superscripts in the same row ($^{a, b}$) or column ($^{1-3}$) indicate that mean values differ significantly (Tukey's test, $p < 0.05$).

The composition of mycoflora changed noticeably during egg storage. Apart from *C. cladosporioides*, the fungal species used for initial eggshell contamination, another two mold genera (*Penicillium* spp. and *Fusarium* spp.) as well as yeasts have also been isolated from experimental eggs (Table 3 and Figure 1).

Table 3. Proportion of mold genera on the eggshell of experimental eggs stored at 11 °C (Group A), 3 °C (Group B) and 20 °C (Group C).

Day	Group A	Group B	Group C
1	C. cladosporioides (100%)	C. cladosporioides (100%)	C. cladosporioides (100%)
7	C. cladosporioides (94%) Penicillium spp. (6%)	C. cladosporioides (100%)	C. cladosporioides (100%)
14	C. cladosporioides (9%) Penicillium spp. (91%)	C. cladosporioides (32%) Penicillium spp. (68%)	C. cladosporioides (20%) Penicillium spp. (80%)
21	C. cladosporioides (34%) Penicillium spp. (33%) Fusarium spp. (33%)	C. cladosporioides (12%) Penicillium spp. (88%)	C. cladosporioides (57%) Penicillium spp. (29%) Yeasts (14%)
28	C. cladosporioides (99%) Penicillium spp. (1%)	C. cladosporioides (100%)	C. cladosporioides (100%)

C.—*Cladosporium*.

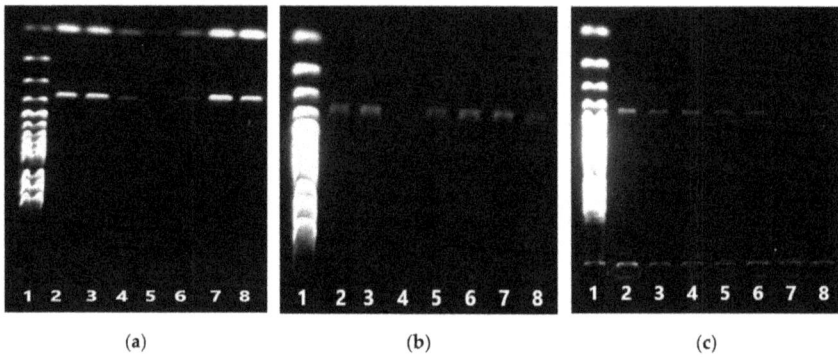

Figure 1. Detection of individual mold genera by PCR: (**a**) *Cladosporium* spp. (87 bp; internal control 370 bp) Line 1: 100 bp ladder standard; Line 2: *Cladosporium cladosporioides* CCM F-348; Lines 3 to 8: isolates of *Cladosporium* spp.; (**b**) *Penicillium* spp. (336 bp) Line 1: 100 bp ladder standard; Line 2: *Penicillium chrysogenum* CCM F-362; Lines 3,5,6,7, and 8: isolates of *Penicillium* spp.; Line 4: non- *Penicillium* spp isolate; (**c**) *Fusarium* spp. (410 bp) Line 1: 100 bp ladder standard; Line 2: *Fusarium graminearun* CCM F-683; Lines 3 to 8: isolates of *Fusarium* spp.

3.2. Growth Characteristics of Cladosporium, Penicillium and Fusarium Species

As can be seen in Table 4, the growth of *C. cladosporioides* and *C. herbarum* on both DRBC and SDA was confirmed 24–72 h later than that of the *Penicillium* and *Fusarium* species used in this study. In addition, all *Penicillium* and *Fusarium* strains showed less intense growth with small colony diameters.

The interactions between the *C. cladosporioides*, *Penicillium* and *Fusarium* species were evaluated after a 120-h cultivation on both DRBC and SDA. The antifungal activity of *C. cladoporioides* was confirmed against *P. chrysogenum*, *P. crustosum* and *P. griseofulvum*. Moreover, mutual inhibition was observed among the four *Penicillium* species tested. On the other hand, the growth of *Fusarium graminearum* was not inhibited by any of the *Penicillium* and *Cladosporium* species tesed in this study (Figure 2).

Table 4. Colony diameters (Ø) of *Cladosporium*, *Penicillium* and *Fusarium* species grown on Dichloran Rose Bengal Chloramphenicol agar (DRBC) and Sabouraud Dextrose Agar (SDA) (mean ± SD).

Fungal Species	Incubation Period (h)				
	24	48	72	96	120
			DRBC (a_w = 0.91) Ø (mm)		
C. cladosporioides CCM F-348	neg	pos$^+$	7.00 ± 0.00	9.67 ± 0.58	12.67 ± 0.58
C. herbarum CCM F-455	neg	neg	pos$^+$	8.33 ± 0.58	11.00 ± 0.00
P. chrysogenum CCM F-362	pos$^+$	8.00 ± 0.00	11.67 ± 0.58	14.33 ± 0.58	18.00 ± 0.00
P. crustosum CCM F-8322	pos$^+$	10.00 ± 0.00	12.00 ± 0.58	16.67 ± 0.58	19.67 ± 0.58
P. griseofulvum CCM F-8006	pos$^+$	8.33 ± 1.25	12.17 ± 1.04	14.67 ± 0.58	17.67 ± 0.58
P. glabrum CCM F-310	pos^{++}	12.00 ± 0.00	16.67 ± 0.58	20.33 ± 0.58	23.67 ± 0.58
F. graminerum CCM F-683	pos$^+$	12.00 ± 0.00	24.67 ± 0.58	25.67 ± 0.58	27.67 ± 1.15
			SDA (a_w = 0.94) Ø (mm)		
C. cladosporioides CCM F-348	pos$^+$	8.67 ± 0.58	12.33 ± 1.15	12.33 ± 1.15	13.00 ± 1.00
C. herbarum CCM F-455	neg	pos+	7.67 ± 0.58	7.67 ± 0.58	10.00 ± 0.00
P. chrysogenum CCM F-8322	pos$^+$	14.67 ± 0.58	20.33 ± 0.58	20.33 ± 0.58	28.67 ± 0.58
P. crustosum CCM F-8322	pos^{++}	13.67 ± 0.58	19.00 ± 0.00	19.00 ± 0.00	25.00 ± 0.00
P. griseofulvum CCM F-8006	pos^{+++}	15.00 ± 0.58	19.33 ± 0.58	19.33 ± 0.58	24.00 ± 0.00
P. glabrum CCM F-310	pos^{+++}	18.33 ± 0.58	27.67 ± 0.58	27.67 ± 0.58	36.67 ± 1.53
F. graminerum CCM F-683	pos$^+$	27.67 ± 1.15	43.00 ± 1.00	43.00 ± 1.00	46.33 ± 1.53

h—hours; neg.—no growth; pos$^+$—growth observed at 10× magnification; pos^{++}—growth observed with the naked eye on the surface of the disk; pos^{+++}—growth observed with the naked eye even around the disk.

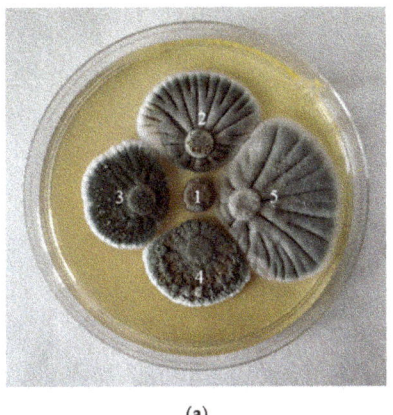
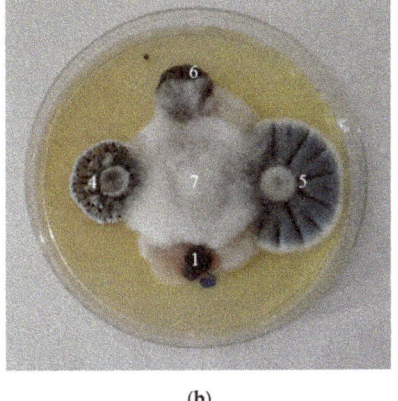

(a) (b)

Figure 2. Antifungal activity of mold species tested in this study: (**a**) *C. cladosporioides* CCM F-348 (1), *P. chrysogenum* CCM F-362 (2), *P. crustosum* CCM F-8322 (3), *P. griseofulvum* CCM F-8006 (4), *P. glabrum* CCM F-310 (5); (**b**) *C. cladosporioides* CCM F-348 (1), *P. griseofulvum* CCM F-8006 (4), *P. glabrum* CCM F-310 (5), *F. graminearum* CCM F-683 (6), *C. herbarum* CCM F-455 (7).

3.3. Effect of Storage Conditions on Egg Quality Parameters

The measurements of selected quality parameters in experimental groups of table eggs are presented in Table 5. Among the five parameters studied, the impact of the storage period was only confirmed in the case of Haugh units and the color of the yolk ($p < 0.05$). As for egg weight, significant differences were observed on Day 21 between experimental Groups B and C ($p < 0.01$). Differences in Haugh units (HU) between experimental groups A and B were only determined on Day 7 ($p < 0.01$). As follows from the results of this study, the most remarkable changes in egg quality were observed when eggs had been stored at laboratory temperature (Group C). Maximum weigh losses were detected between Day 7 and Day 14 of the experiment with an average value of 3.5%. In group C eggs, Haugh units decreased continuously within the storage period. At the end of experiment (Day 28), most eggs had to be downgraded to Grade B.

Table 5. Egg quality parameters in three experimental groups of table eggs (A–C) during storage (mean ± SD).

Parameter	Group	Storage Period [Days]				ANOVA [p Values]	
		7	14	21	28	Impact of Storage Conditions	Impact of Storage Period
Egg weight [g]	A	62.47 ± 3.07 a1	60.35 ± 3.55 a1	60.37 ± 2.37 a12	62.80 ± 1.44 a1	$p < 0.01$	$p > 0.05$
	B	62.25 ± 1.55 a1	62.05 ± 0.85 a1	62.00 ± 0.53 a1	62.43 ± 3.29 a1		
	C	62.43 ± 0.61 a1	56.80 ± 4.20 a1	57.00 ± 1.60 a2	59.15 ± 1.55 a1		
Eggshell firmness [kgf]	A	4.33 ± 0.18 a1	4.67 ± 0.65 a1	4.72 ± 0.29 a1	4.99 ± 0.36 a1	$p > 0.05$	$p > 0.05$
	B	3.99 ± 2.16 a1	4.70 ± 0.38 a1	2.60 ± 2.49 a1	5.01 ± 0.43 a1		
	C	5.10 ± 0.22 a1	4.08 ± 2.40 a1	5.13 ± 0.33 a1	5.83 ± 0.96 a1		
Haugh units [HU]	A	86.87 ± 2.78 a1	83.65 ± 5.35 a1	78.57 ± 6.49 a1	78.27 ± 7.51 a1	$p < 0.01$	$p < 0.05$
	B	70.05 ± 5.05 a2	84.40 ± 2.90 a1	69.93 ± 8.56 a1	70.77 ± 12.64 a1		
	C	78.10 ± 4.65 a12	74.85 ± 3.15 a1	70.90 ± 2.40 ab1	66.75 ± 0.25 b1		
Yolk color	A	10.00 ± 0.00 a1	7.00 ± 3.00 a1	9.00 ± 1.00 a1	7.00 ± 2.65 a1	$p > 0.05$	$p < 0.05$
	B	10.00 ± 0.00 a1	10.33 ± 0.58 a1	7.67 ± 2.31 a1	9.67 ± 1.15 a1		
	C	10.00 ± 0.00 a1	9.33 ± 0.58 a1	9.00 ± 1.00 ab1	6.67 ± 1.53 b1		
Grade of quality	A	AA a1	AA a1	AA a1	A–AA a1	$p > 0.05$	$p > 0.05$
	B	A–AA a1	A–AA a1	A–AA a1	B–AA a1		
	C	AA a1	A–AA a1	B–AA a1	B–A a1		

Different superscripts in the same row (a, b) or column (1,2) indicate that mean values differ significantly (Tukey's test, $p < 0.05$).

3.4. Statistical Analysis

Statistical analysis of results achieved in this study is shown in Table 6. The Pearson's correlation matrix demonstrates reciprocal correlations between individual quality parameters studied in experimental groups of table eggs. Significant differences are highlighted in bold. Correlations between the following parameters at the level of $p < 0.05$ can be seen in this table: eggshell firmness and the count of molds on the shell surface ($r = -0.385$), Haugh units and quality grades of table eggs ($r = 0.717$), Haugh units and relative humidity ($r = 0.440$), yolk color and the count of molds present in the yolk ($r = -0.345$), egg weight and storage temperature ($r = -0.490$), egg weight and relative humidity ($r = 0.334$), the count of molds in the egg white and in the egg yolk ($r = 0.748$), grade of quality and relative humidity ($r = 0.351$), storage temperature and relative humidity ($r = -0.402$), storage temperature and dew point temperature ($r = 0.816$).

Table 6. Pearson's correlation matrix for egg quality parameters (significant differences are highlighted in bold).

Parameter	Shell Firmness	Haugh Units	Yolk Color	Egg Weight	CFU/ Eggshell *	CFU/g Albumen *	CFU/g Yolk *	Grade of Quality	Temperature	Relative Humidity	Dew Point
Shell firmness		0.188	0.078	−0.101	**−0.385**	−0.204	−0.242	0.074	0.267	−0.136	0.199
Haugh units	0.188		0.206	0.109	0.108	0.054	−0.031	**0.717**	−0.079	**0.440**	0.205
Yolk color	0.078	0.206		0.215	0.046	−0.252	**−0.345**	0.233	−0.154	−0.155	−0.249
Egg weight	−0.101	0.109	0.215		−0.146	−0.148	−0.239	0.136	**−0.490**	**0.334**	−0.308
CFU/eggshell *	**−0.385**	0.108	0.046	−0.146		0.031	0.209	0.073	−0.130	−0.030	−0.147
CFU/g albumen *	−0.204	0.054	−0.252	−0.148	0.031		**0.748**	0.148	−0.038	0.148	0.067
CFU/g yolk *	−0.242	−0.031	−0.345	−0.239	0.209	**0.748**		−0.075	−0.011	0.054	0.009
Grade of quality	0.074	**0.717**	0.233	0.136	0.073	0.148	−0.075		−0.135	**0.351**	0.084
Temperature	0.267	−0.079	−0.154	**−0.490**	−0.130	−0.038	−0.011	−0.135		**−0.402**	**0.816**
Relative humidity	−0.136	**0.440**	−0.155	**0.334**	−0.030	0.148	0.054	**0.351**	**−0.402**		0.189
Dew point	0.199	0.205	−0.249	−0.308	−0.147	0.067	0.009	0.084	**0.816**	0.189	

CFU colony forming unit. * number of molds.

The MFA statistical method was applied to the data of microbial and quality parameters of experimental eggs and parameters of storage conditions, whereas storage conditions and storage period were set as the main qualitative factors. The results of MFA show five selected components, which explain 77.78% of the total variation in the dataset. The first dimension (Dim1) explains 20.78%, dimension 2 (Dim2) 18.03%, dimension 3 (Dim3) 16.05%, dimension 4 (Dim4) 12.54% and dimension 5 (Dim5) 9.34% of variation.

The contribution of the data analysed in Dim1 was related to parameters of storage conditions (39.32%, r = 0.95). The first two dimensions explained a total of 38.81% of variance (see Figure 3). The highest contribution in Dim1 included relative humidity (r = 0.51), dew point temperature (r = −0.70) and storage temperature (r = −0.95). Dim2 was characterized by the contribution of the effect of storage conditions (43.40%, r = 0.92) on the analyzed parameters.

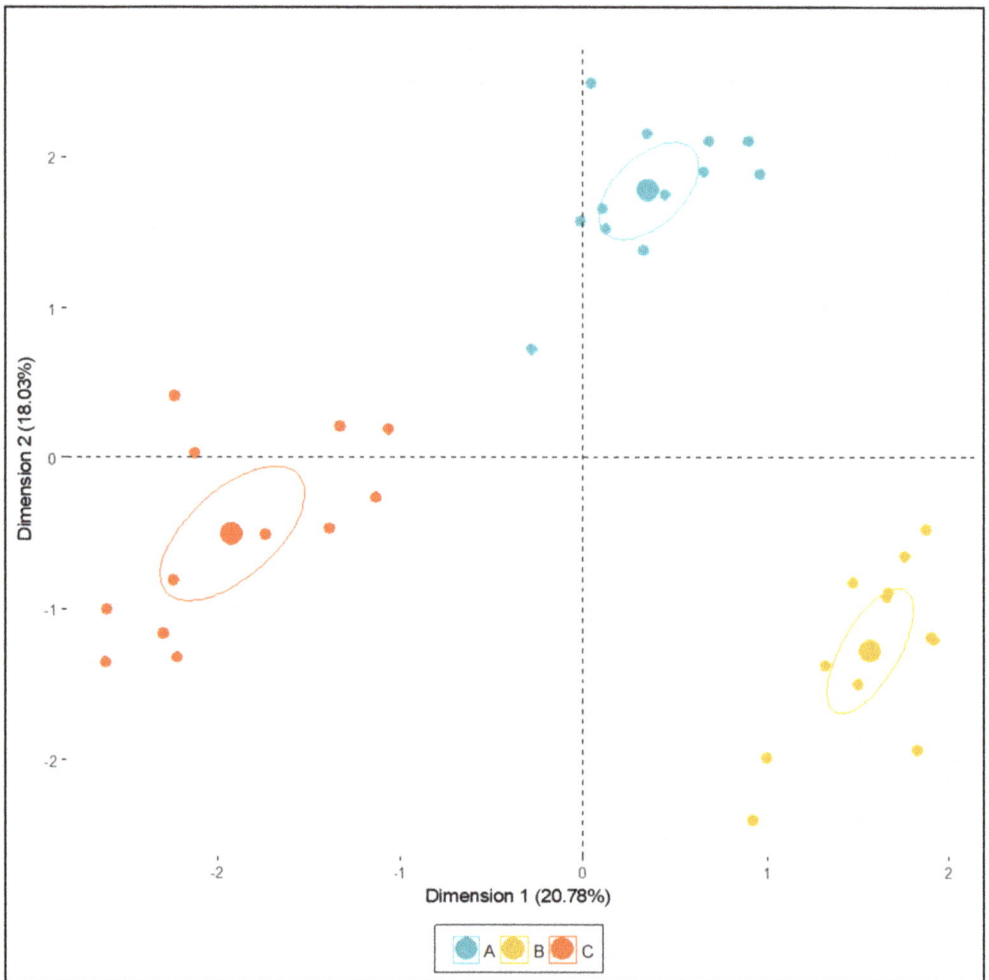

Figure 3. Plot of individuals in the first and second extracted dimension under different storage conditions. A—table eggs stored at average temperature of (11.43 ± 0.20) °C, relative humidity of (79.00 ± 2.94)% and the dew point of (7.90 ± 0.47) °C. B—table eggs stored at average temperature of (3.33 ± 1.1) °C, relative humidity of (57.76 ± 5.30)% and the dew point of (−4.25 ± 1.96) °C. C—table eggs stored at average temperature of (20.60 ± 1.04) °C, relative humidity of (43.55 ± 5.93)% and the dew point of (7.60 ± 2.39) °C.

Parameters in the first two dimension were correlated on statistical significant level α < 0.05 (see Figure 4). Dim3 was related mostly to the microbial parameters of experimental groups of eggs (44.35%, r = 0.89). Correlation coefficients for microbial parameters in Dim3 were determined as follows: CFU in the egg yolk (r = 0.77), CFU in the egg white (r = 0.71) and CFU in the eggshell (r = 0.54). Dim4 shows relations mainly in quality parameters of experimental egg groups (23.06%, r = 0.66). In Dim4, there were statistically significant correlations for yolk color (r = 0.61) and egg quality grade (r = 0.37). Dim5 explains mostly the effect of storage period on monitored egg parameters (88.53%, r = 0.98).

From the results obtained by MFA, it follows that the effects of storage conditions on experimental eggs were statistically significant. The MFA method showed differences between experimental egg groups A, B and C, which were visualized in different segments of individual plots (see Figures 3 and 4).

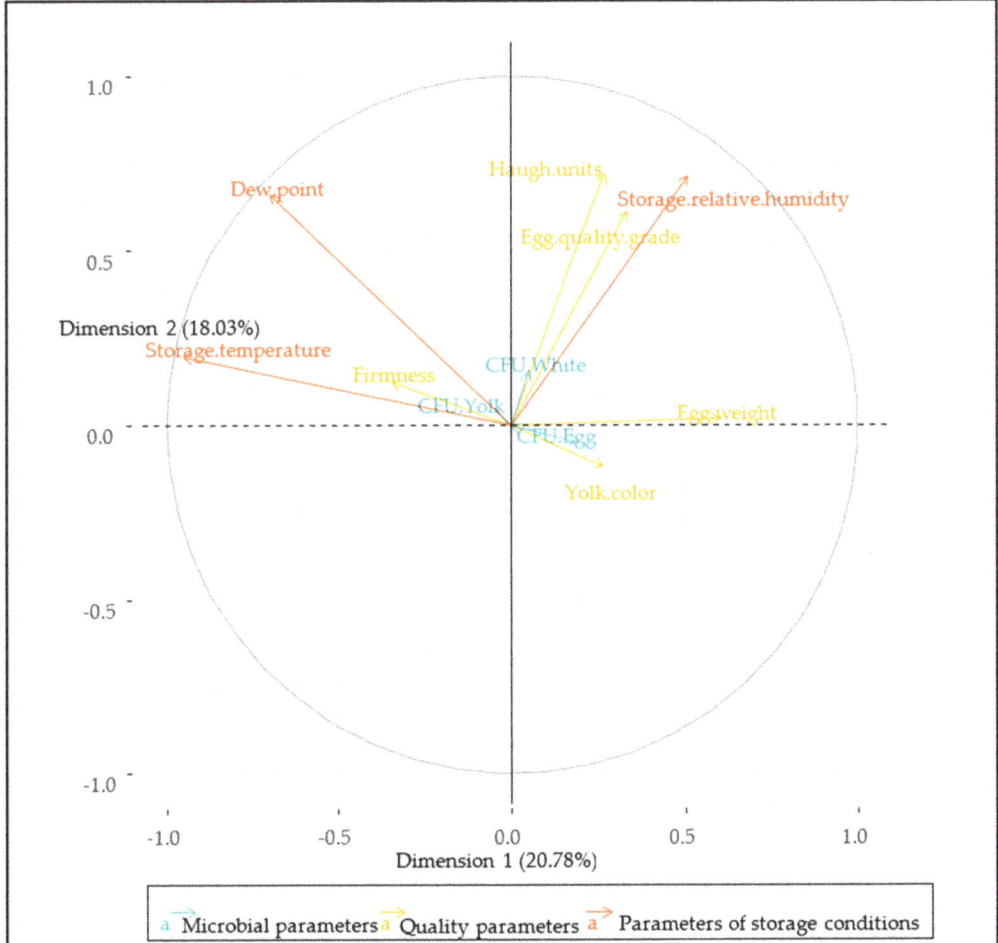

Figure 4. Correlation plot of variables in the first and second extracted dimension under different storage conditions.

4. Discussion

It is a well-known fact that the egg quality and the growth of contaminating mycoflora on the shell surface depend mainly on storage conditions. The aim of the present study was to examine the interaction between the storage time, *C. cladosporioides* contamination and their effect on the quality of table eggs.

Results of previous studies performed at the Department of Food Hygiene, Technology and Safety of the University of Veterinary Medicine and Pharmacy in Košice have demonstrated that the genus *Cladosporium* is one of the most common type of mold on the eggshells in egg storage facilities [34,35]. Due to tolerance to low temperatures, *C. cladosporioides* is able to colonize refrigerated food products as well as refrigerator interiors [36]. In this study, egg storage temperatures were chosen in accordance with Commission Regulation No 589/2008 [37], with the minimum limited to 5 °C. As the storage temperatures ensure an optimum egg quality within the 28 days, most egg producers recommend storing the eggs at temperatures between 5 °C and 18 °C.

The results of this study demonstrate that the average counts of molds on/in the eggs remained practically unchanged across the entire storage period. However, noticeable changes were observed in the composition of mycoflora during egg storage. Apart from *C. cladosporioides*, the fungal species used for initial eggshell contamination, the presence of another two mold genera (*Penicillium* spp. and *Fusarium* spp.) as well as yeasts have also been detected in the experimental eggs.

Fluctuating air humidity results in a transient water supply affecting both spore germination and fungal growth. Wu and Wong [38] reported growth retardation of *C. cladosporioides* spores exposed to daily cycles with various combinations of wet and dry periods. The longer the phase of growth retardation, the higher the intracellular concentration of hydrogen peroxide. Thus, the fluctuating air humidity may result in slowing growth of *C. cladosporioides* and subsequent oxidative stress.

Visible growth of either *C. cladosporioides* or the other mold genera was not detected on/in experimental table eggs across the entire period of this study. This result could probably be explained by the variable germination ability of spores, which differs considerably depending on environmental conditions [39] and low relative humidity during egg storage. As for *C. cladosporioides*, the minimum values of available water (a_w) required for spore germination range between 0.85 and 0.91 and those for sporulation between 0.87 and 0.95 [20]. Mold development on the shell surface can also be facilitated by low temperatures, provided that the relative humidity is higher than 90% [19]. The spores of *Penicillium* spp. germinate from 0.79 a_w (*P. piceum*) to 0.83 a_w (*P. roqueforti*) [40].

The isolates of *Penicillium* spp. were dominant on experimental days when the maximum relative humidity and dew point temperature were observed. The proportion of penicillia on these days varied from 68 to 91% depending on the particular experimental group. The results of this study indicate that *Penicillium* and *Fusarium* species grow faster at higher a_w (0.91–0.94). Thus, they may pose a risk to the consumer in the case of eggshell contamination. While the adverse effects of *C. cladosporioides* metabolites are still under investigation [41], the toxicity of secondary metabolites produced by *Penicillium* and *Fusarium* species has already been reliably confirmed [42–44]. Among the hundreds of identified mycotoxins endangering human or animal health, aflatoxins, ochratoxin A, patulin and fusarial mycotoxins (fumonisins, zearalenon and nivalenol/deoxynivalenol) are of greatest concern [45]. *P. verrucosum* and *P. nordicum* have been recognized as major producers of ochratoxin A [46]. The presence of *P. verrucosum* was also detected among fungal contaminants of table eggs [47], indicating a possible risk of egg contamination with ochratoxin A. *Fusarium* sp. is reported to produce a number of mycotoxins, including trichothecens such as deoxynivalenol (DON), nivalenol (NIV), T-2 and HT-2 toxins, as well as zearalenon (ZEN) and fumonisins [48]. As reported by Tomczyk et al. [49], contamination of table eggs with *F. culmorum* has resulted in the presence of DON, 3-AcDON and NIV in the egg contents. Growth of *Aspergillus flavus* on the eggshell may lead to contamination of egg contents with aflatoxins [50].

The genus *Penicillium* is quite common in table eggs [47]. The results of a Nigerian study confirmed the presence of this fungus in 82.5% of sampled eggs [16]. The combination of appropriate environmental conditions and a poor level of hygiene may lead to proliferation of microorganisms including molds [18,49,51].

The growth of competetive mycoflora can also be affected by mutual interactions [52]. In this study, antifungal activity of *C. cladosporioides* against *P. chrysogenum*, *P. crustosum* and *P. griseofulvum*, as well as mutual inhibition among *Penicillium* species tested, has been confirmed. *C. cladosporioides* belongs to xerophilic and psychrophilic molds which are able to produce at least three metabolites (cladosporin, isocladosporin and 5′-hydroxyasperentin) and their derivates, showing antifungal activity against pathogenic mold genera including *Aspergillus* spp., *Penicillium* spp., *Phomopsis viticola*, *Colletotrichum acutatum*, *Colletotrichum fragariae*, *Colletotrichum gloeosporioides* [41,53].

The *Penicillium* genus is known to produce bioactive molecules with a strong antifungal effect [54–57]. Mutual antifungal activity against at least one of the toxigenic *P. echinulatum* and *P. commune* strains was already confirmed in 85 strains of 17 *Penicillium* species, including *P. chrysogenum* *P. crustosum*, and *P. griseofulvum* [57].

As follows from the results of this study, storage conditions can significantly influence egg quality parameters. Based on Haugh units, experimental eggs were classified into three quality grades (AA, A and B). In extra fresh eggs (AA grade), the HU were above 72. Numerous factors are reported to influence HU quality grades, and among them, storage temperature and storage period are of greatest concern [58]. In this study, a continuous decrease in both HU and yolk color was observed during the egg storage period in all the three experimental groups ($p < 0.05$). On Day 7, the differences between experimental groups A and B were significant ($p < 0.01$). As for egg weight, noticeable changes were confirmed on Day 21 between experimental groups B and C ($p < 0.01$). The most significant decrease in freshness was observed in group C experimental eggs stored at temperatures between (20.00 ± 0.86) °C and (22.09 ± 0.13) °C and air humidity between $(40.75 \pm 3.42)\%$ and $(45.47 \pm 1.49)\%$. At the end of the storage period (Day 28), the following egg quality parameters were observed in Group C: egg weight (59.15 ± 1.55) g, HU (66.75 ± 0.25), yolk color (6.67 ± 1.53) and quality grade (A–B). Other studies reported similar effects of storage period and storage temperature on the egg quality parameters [50,55–63]. Prolonged storage period has resulted in a gradual decrease in the egg weight, HU and yolk color, this being less significant at low storage temperatures (0–5 °C) and more noticeable at higher temperatures (20–29 °C).

Fedde et al. [59] found out that the quality parameters of eggs stored for 9 weeks in the cold were simiar to those observed for eggs stored at room temperature for 3 weeks. Refrigeration storage at (4 ± 2) °C is able to maintain safety and nutritive value of table eggs for approximately 4–5 weeks [60–63]. A decrease in HU from 91.4 to 76.3 was reported for eggs stored at 5 °C for 10 days [64]. An increase in storage temperature to 29 °C has lead to significant weight losses (1.74% within 5 days and 3.67% within 10 days) accompanied with a decrease in HU from 87.62 to 60.92 [65]. Similar results were also obtained in other studies [66,67]. The decrease in HU may result from the escape of carbon dioxide from the egg white, leading to a watery consistency and lower height of the thick albumen—the two parameters considered in HU calculation [68].

Changes in yolk color result from aging of the yolk membrane. Water from the egg albumen is absorbed by the yolk, where it dilutes the yolk pigments and makes the color paler. Long-term egg storage may also result in the penetration of albumen proteins into the egg yolk, causing a decrease in yolk color as well [69]. Elevated storage temperatures accelerate the destruction of the protein structure in both the thick albumen and the vitelline membrane [70]. All the above-mentioned changes have been observed even after a 2-day storage of table eggs at 29 °C [65].

Loss in egg weight is more commonly associated with water evaporation than with the escape of carbon dioxide (CO_2), ammonia, nitrogen and hydrogen sulphide through the shell pores [64]. More significant weight losses are reported for eggs stored at higher ambient temperature and lower relative humidity [71]. In this study, the most noticeable weight losses were observed in Group C experimental eggs stored for 28 days at the highest temperature (20 °C) and lowest relative humidity (45%). Moreover, the results of this study revealed a close reciprocal correlation between relative air humidity and eggshell firmness, where firmness was significantly reduced with an increase in air humidity in the egg storage room. As reported by Tyler and Geake [72], moisture in the air makes the eggshell weaker. However, the shell regains its firmness after drying in air.

5. Conclusions

Despite of initial eggshell contamination with spore suspension of *C. cladosporioides*, the results of this study did not confirm any visible growth of molds on/in table eggs stored for 28 days at three different temperatures (3 °C, 11 °C and 20 °C) and relative humidity between 45 to 80%. As demonstrated in this study, high relative air humidity in the egg storage room reduced the growth of *C. cladosporioides*, probably due to oxidative stress resulting from the previous fluctuating humidity values, and favored the growth of *Penicillium* spp.

Comparison of growth characteristics among seven fungal species (*C. cladosporioides* CCM F-348, *C. herbarum* CCM F-455, *P. chrysogenum* CCM F-362, *P. crustosum* CCM F-8322, *P. griseofulvum* CCM F-8006, *P. glabrum* CCM F-310, *F. graminearum* CCM F-683) on the selective culture media (DRBC and SDA) has demonstrated that both *Cladosporium* species grow 24–72 h later than *Penicillium* and *Fusarium* species on the eggshell surface. Furthermore, the results of this study confirmed the inhibition activity of *C. cladosporiorides* CCM F-348 against four *Penicillium* species tested but not against *F. graminerum* CCM F-683. Both *Penicillium* and *Fusarium* species showed more intense growth with larger colony diameters on the surface of the eggshell at high values of relative air humidity, thus increasing the risk to consumers due to possible contamination of egg contents with mycotoxins.

Based on the results obtained, it can be concluded that the most appropriate temperature for egg storage is 11 °C, and the optimum range of relative humidity lies between 75% and 81%. Table eggs stored under such conditions maintained their grade of quality within the entire storage period of 28 days. The other quality parameters also remained unaffected, except for yolk color, which declined steadily during egg storage. In terms of egg quality, the least appropriate conditions for egg storage are temperatures close to 20 °C. Due to weight loss, most eggs stored at this temperature had to be downgraded at the end of the shelf life period. In addition, increased numbers of fungal spores on the egg surface adversely affected the firmness of the eggshell as well as color of the yolk. The results of this study have demonstrated that storage conditions are crucial for maintaining egg quality and mycological safety of table eggs for consumers.

Author Contributions: P.J. and M.P.; methodology, P.J.; software, B.S.; formal analysis, M.P.; investigation, S.D. and I.R.; data curation, B.S.; Writing—Original draft preparation, P.J.; Writing—Review and editing, M.P.; visualization, I.K.; supervision, J.N.; project administration, P.J.; funding acquisition, S.M. All authors have read and agreed to the published version of the manuscript.

Funding: This research was funded by the Operational Program Integrated Infrastructure within the project: Demand-driven research for the sustainable and inovative food, Drive4SIFood 313011V336, cofinanced by the European Regional Development Fund (70%) and by the Cultural and Educational Grant Agency of the Ministry of Education, Science, Research and Sport of the Slovak Republic and the Slovak Academy of Sciences KEGA 013UVLF-4/2021(30%).

Institutional Review Board Statement: Not applicable.

Informed Consent Statement: Not applicable.

Data Availability Statement: The data presented in this study are available on request from the corresponding author.

Conflicts of Interest: The authors declare no conflict of interest.

References

1. Aihara, M.; Tanaka, T.; Takatori, K. *Cladosporium* as the main fungal contaminant of locations in dwelling environments. *Biocontrol Sci.* **2001**, *6*, 49–52. [CrossRef]
2. Ohta, T.; Park, B.J.; Aihara, M.; Ri, N.; Saito, T.; Sawada, T.; Takatori, K. Morphological significance of *Cladosporium* contaminants on materials and utensils in contact with food. *Biocontrol Sci.* **2006**, *11*, 55–60. [CrossRef]
3. Aira, M.J.; Rodríguez-Rajo, F.J.; Fernández-González, M.; Seijo, C.; Elvira-Rendueles, B.; Gutiérrez-Bustillo, M.; Abreu, I.; Pérez-Sánchez, E.; Oliveira, M.; Recio, M.; et al. *Cladosporium* airborne spore incidence in the environmental quality of the Iberian Peninsula. *Grana* **2012**, *51*, 293–304. [CrossRef]
4. Bensch, K.; Braun, U.; Groenewald, J.Z.; Crous, P.W. The genus *Cladosporium*. *Stud. Mycol.* **2012**, *72*, 1–401. [CrossRef]
5. Ogórek, R.; Lejman, A.; Pusz, W.; Miłuch, A.; Miodyńska, P. Characteristics and taxonomy of *Cladosporium* fungi. *Mikologia Lekarska* **2012**, *19*, 80–85.
6. Temperini, C.V.; Franchi, M.L.; Rozo, M.E.B.; Grecob, M.; Pardo, A.G.; Pose, G.P. Diversity and abundance of airborne fungal spores in a rural cold dry desert environment in Argentinean Patagonia. *Sci. Total Environ.* **2019**, *665*, 513–520. [CrossRef]
7. Bensch, K.; Groenewald, J.Z.; Meijer, M.; Dijksterhuis, J.; Jurjević, Ž.; Andersen, B.; Houbraken, J.; Crous, P.W.; Samson, R.A. *Cladosporium* species in indoor environments. *Stud. Mycol.* **2018**, *89*, 177–301. [CrossRef]
8. Bensch, K.; Groenewald, J.Z.; Braun, U.; Dijksterhuis, J.; de Jesús Yánez-Morales, M.; Crous, P.W. Common but different: The expanding realm of *Cladosporium*. *Stud. Mycol.* **2015**, *82*, 23–74. [CrossRef]
9. Marin-Felix, Y.; Groenewald, J.Z.; Cai, L.; Chen, Q.; Marincowitz, S.; Barnes, I.; Bensch, K.; Braun, U.; Camporesi, E.; Damm, U.; et al. Genera of phytopathogenic fungi: GOPHY 1. *Stud. Mycol.* **2017**, *86*, 99–216. [CrossRef]
10. Costanzo, N.; Rodolfi, M.; Musarella, R.; Ceniti, C.; Santoro, A.; Britti, D.; Casalinuovo, F. Microbial quality evaluation of grated cheese samples collected at retail level in Calabria (Italy). *J. Food Saf.* **2018**, *38*, e12530. [CrossRef]
11. Biango-Daniels, M.N.; Hodge, K.T. Sea salts as a potential source of food spoilage fungi. *Food Microbiol.* **2018**, *69*, 89–95. [CrossRef] [PubMed]
12. Regecová, I.; Pipová, M.; Jevinová, P.; Demjanová, S.; Semjon, B. Quality and mycobiota composition of stored eggs. *Ital. J. Food Sci.* **2020**, *32*, 540–561. [CrossRef]
13. Vlčková, J.; Tůmová, E.; Ketta, M.; Englmaierová, M.; Chodová, D. Effect of housing system and age of laying hens on eggshell quality, microbial contamination, and penetration of microorganisms into eggs. *Czech J. Anim. Sci.* **2018**, *63*, 51–60. [CrossRef]
14. De Reu, K.; Messens, W.; Heyndrickx, M.; Rodenburg, T.B.; Uyttendaele, M.; Herman, L. Bacterial contamination of table eggs and the influence of housing systems. *World's Poult. Sci. J.* **2008**, *64*, 5–19. [CrossRef]
15. Salem, R.M.; El-Kaseh, R.M.; El-Diaty, E.M. A study on the fungal contamination and prevalence of aflatoxins and some antibiotic residues in table eggs. *Arab. J. Biotechnol.* **2009**, *12*, 65–71.
16. Obi, C.N.; Igbokwe, A.J. Microbiological analyses of freshly laid and stored domestic poultry eggs in selected poultry farms in Umuahia, Abia State, Nigeria. *Res. J. Biol. Sci.* **2009**, *4*, 1297–1303. [CrossRef]
17. Mounam, M.A.W.A.; Al-Ameed, A.I.; Al-Gburi, N.M. A study of moulds contamination of, table eggs in Baghdad city. *J. Genet. Environ. Resour. Conserv.* **2014**, *2*, 107–111.
18. Salihu, M.D.; Garba, B.; Isah, Y. Evaluation of microbial contents of table eggs at retail outlets in Sokoto metropolis, Nigeria. *Sok. J. Vet. Sci.* **2015**, *13*, 22–28. [CrossRef]
19. Tančinová, D.; Kačániová, M.; Felšőciová, S.; Mašková, Z. *Mikrobiológia Potravín*, 1st ed.; Slovak University of Agriculture: Nitra, Slovakia, 2017; p. 239. ISBN 978-80-552-1642-3.
20. Aihara, M.; Tanaka, T.; Takatori, T.O.K. Effect of temperature and water activity on the growth of *Cladosporium sphaerospermum* and *Cladosporium cladosporioides*. *Biocontrol. Sci.* **2002**, *7*, 193–196. [CrossRef]
21. Sørhaug, T. Yeasts and molds. Spoilage molds in dairy products. In *Encyclopedia of Dairy Sciences*, 2nd ed.; Fuquay, J.W., Ed.; Academic Press: Cambridge, MA, USA, 2011; pp. 780–784, ISBN 978-0-12-374407-4.
22. Cupáková, Š.; Karpíšková, R.; Necidová, L. *Mikrobiologie Potravin. Praktická Cvičení*, 2nd ed.; University of Veterinary and Pharmaceutical Sciences: Brno, Czech Republic, 2010; pp. 30–31, ISBN 978-80-7305-126-6.
23. ISO. *Microbiology of the Food Chain. Preparation of Test Samples, Initial Suspensions and Decimal Dilutions for Microbiological Examination. Part. 1: General Rules for the Preparation of the Initial Suspension and Decimal Dilutions*; ISO 6887-1:2017; Slovak Standards Institute: Bratislava, Slovakia, 2017.
24. ISO. *Microbiology of Food and Animal Feeding Stuffs. Horizontal Method for the Enumeration of Yeasts and Molds. Part. 2: Colony Count Technique in Products with Water Activity less than or Equal to 0.95*; ISO 21527-2:2008; Slovak Standards Institute: Bratislava, Slovakia, 2010.
25. Frisvad, J.C.; Samson, R.A. Polyphasic taxonomy of *Penicillium* subgenus *Penicillium*. A guide to identification of food and air-borne terverticillate penicillia and their mycotoxins. *Stud. Mycol.* **2004**, *49*, 1–175.
26. Tančinová, D.; Mašková, Z.; Felšőciová, S.; Dovičičová, M.; Barboráková, Z. *Úvod do Potravinárskej Mykológie*, 1st ed.; Slovak University of Agriculture: Nitra, Slovakia, 2012; pp. 143–244, ISBN 97-880-5520-753-7.
27. Pedersen, L.H.; Skouboe, P.; Boysen, M.; Souleb, J.; Rossen, L. Detection of *Penicillium* species in complex food samples using the polymerase chain reaction. *Int. J. Food Microbiol.* **1997**, *35*, 169–177. [CrossRef]
28. Abd-Elsalam, K.A.; Aly, I.N.; Abdel-Satar, M.A.; Khalil, M.S.; Verreet, J.A. PCR identification of *Fusarium* genus based on nuclear ribosomal-DNA sequence data. *Afr. J. Biotechnol.* **2003**, *2*, 82–85. [CrossRef]

29. Zeng, Q.Y.; Westermark, S.O.; Lestanderb, R.; Wang, X.R. Detection and quantification of *Cladosporium* in aerosols by real-time PCR. *J. Environ. Monit.* **2006**, *8*, 153–160. [CrossRef]
30. R Core Team. *A Language and Environment for Statistical Computing*; Version 3.5.1.; Foundation for Statistical Computing: Vienna, Austria, 2018; Available online: https://www.R-project.org/ (accessed on 9 May 2019).
31. Sebastien, L.; Josse, J.; Husson, F. FactoMineR: An R package for multivariate analysis. *J. Stat. Soft.* **2008**, *25*, 1–18. [CrossRef]
32. Kassambara, A.; Mundt, F. Factoextra: Extract and Visualize the Results of Multivariate Data Analysis. In *R Package Version 1.0.5.*; Foundation for Statistical Computing: Vienna, Austria, 2007; Available online: https://CRAN.R-project.org/package=factoextra (accessed on 9 May 2019).
33. Semjon, B.; Král, M.; Pospiech, M.; Reitznerová, A.; Maľová, J.; Tremlová, B.; Dudriková, E. Application of multiple factor analysis for the descriptive sensory evaluation and instrumental measurements of bryndza cheese as affected by vacuum packaging. *Int. J. Food Prop.* **2018**, *21*, 1508–1522. [CrossRef]
34. Danková, M. The Effect of Temperature and Packing on the Contamination of Chicken Eggs with Micromycetes. Master's Thesis, University of Veterinary Medicine and Pharmacy, Košice, Slovakia, 2017.
35. Ševčíková, P. Impact of Farming Method on the Contamination of Eggs with Microscopic Filamentous Fungi. Master's Thesis, University of Veterinary Medicine and Pharmacy, Košice, Slovakia, 2017.
36. Altunatmaz, S.S.; Issa, G.; Aydin, A. Detection of airborne psychrotrophic bacteria and fungi in food storage refrigerators. *Braz. J. Microbiol.* **2012**, *43*, 1436–1443. [CrossRef] [PubMed]
37. Commission Regulation (EC) No. 589/2008 of 23 June 2008 Laying Down Detailed Rules for Implementing Council Regulation (EC) No. 1234/2007 as Regards Marketing Standards for Eggs. Available online: https://eur-lex.europa.eu/LexUriServ/LexUriServ.do?uri=OJ:L:2008:163:0006:0023:EN:PDF (accessed on 20 October 2020).
38. Wu, H.; Wong, J.W.C. The role of oxidative stress in the growth of the indoor mould *Cladosporium cladosporioides* under water dynamics. *Indoor Air* **2019**, *30*, 117–125. [CrossRef]
39. Osherov, N.; May, G.S. The molecular mechanisms of conidial germination. *FEMS Microbiol. Lett.* **2001**, *199*, 153–160. [CrossRef]
40. Magan, N.; Lacey, J. Effect of temperature and pH on water relations of field and storage fungi. *Trans. Br. Mycol. Soc.* **1984**, *82*, 71–81. [CrossRef]
41. Wang, X.; Radwan, M.M.; Taráwneh, A.H.; Gao, J.; Wedge, D.E.; Rosa, L.H.; Cutler, H.G.; Cutler, S.J. Antifungal activity against plant pathogens of metabolites from the endophytic fungus *Cladosporium cladosporioides*. *J. Agric. Food Chem.* **2013**, *19*, 4551–4555. [CrossRef]
42. Frisvad, J.C.; Thrane, U.; Samson, R.A.; Pitt, J.I. Important mycotoxins and the fungi which produce them. *Adv. Food Mycol.* **2006**, *571*, 3–31. [CrossRef]
43. Smith, M.C.; Madec, S.; Coton, E.; Hymery, N. Natural co-occurrence of mycotoxins in foods and feeds and their in vitro combined toxicological effects. *Toxins* **2016**, *8*, 94. [CrossRef]
44. Abbas, M. Co-occurrence of mycotoxins and its detoxification strategies. In *Mycotoxins—Impact and Management Strategies*; Njobeh, P.B., Francois Stepman, F., Eds.; IntechOpen: London, UK, 2019; pp. 91–107. [CrossRef]
45. Milićević, D.R.; Škrinjar, M.; Baltić, T. Real and perceived risks for mycotoxin contamination in foods and feeds: Challenges for food safety control. *Toxins* **2010**, *2*, 572–592. [CrossRef] [PubMed]
46. Perrone, G.; Susca, A. Penicillium species and their associated mycotoxins. In *Mycotoxigenic Fungi*; Chapter 5; Springer: Cham, Switzerland, 2016; pp. 107–119. [CrossRef]
47. Demjanová, S.; Jevinová, P.; Pipová, M.; Regecová, I. Identification of *Penicillium verrucosum*, *Penicillium commune*, and *Penicillium crustosum* isolated from chicken eggs. *Processes* **2021**, *9*, 53. [CrossRef]
48. Nesic, K.; Ivanovic, S.; Nesic, V. Fusarial toxins: Secondary metabolites of *Fusarium* fungi. *Rev. Environ. Contam. Toxicol.* **2013**, *228*, 101–120. [CrossRef]
49. Tomczyk, Ł.; Stępień, Ł.; Urbaniak, M.; Szablewski, T.; Cegielska-Radziejewska, R.; Stuper-Szablewska, K. Characterisation of the mycobiota on the shell surface of table eggs acquired from different egg-laying hen breeding systems. *Toxins* **2018**, *10*, 293. [CrossRef]
50. El Malt, L.M. Assesment of the microbial quality and aflatoxins content in poultry farms eggs sold in Qena city—Upper Egypt. *Assiut Vet. Med. J.* **2015**, *61*, 141–151.
51. Mansour, A.F.A.; Zayed, A.F.; Basha, O.A.A. Contamination of the shell and internal content of table eggs with some pathogens during different storage periods. *Assiut Vet. Med. J.* **2015**, *61*, 8–15.
52. Morón-Ríos, A.; Gómez-Cornelio, S.; Ortega-Morales, B.O.; De la Rosa-García, S.; Partida-Martínez, L.P.; Quintana, P.; Alayo-Gamboa1, J.A.; Cappello-Garcia, S.; González-Gómez, S. Interactions between abundant fungal species influence the fungal community assemblage on limestone. *PLoS ONE* **2017**, *12*, e0188443. [CrossRef]
53. Scott, P.M.; Walbeek, W.V.; Maclean, W.M. Cladosporin, a new antifungal metabolite from *Cladosporium cladosporioides*. *J. Antibiot.* **1971**, *24*, 747–755. [CrossRef]
54. Nicoletti, R.; Stefano, M.D.; Stefano, S.D.; Trincone, A.; Marziano, F. Antagonism against *Rhizoctonia solani* and fungitoxic metabolite production by some *Penicillium* isolates. *Mycopathologia* **2004**, *158*, 465–474. [CrossRef] [PubMed]
55. Khokhar, I.; Mukhtar, I.; Mushtaq, S. Antifungal effect of *Penicillium* metabolites against some fungi. *Arch. Phytopathol. Pflanzenschutz.* **2011**, *44*, 1347–1351. [CrossRef]

56. Boutheina, M.T.; Abdallah Rania, A.B.; Nawaim, A.; Mejda, D.R. Antifungal potential of extracellular metabolites from *Penicillium* spp. and *Aspergillus* spp. Naturally Associated to Potato against *Fusarium* species Causing Tuber Dry Rot. *J. Microb. Biochem. Technol.* **2017**, *9*, 181–190. [CrossRef]
57. Acosta, R.; Rodríguez-Martín, A.; Martín, A.; Núñez, F.; Asensio, M.A. Selection of antifungal protein-producing molds from dry-cured meat products. *Inter. J. Food Microbiol.* **2009**, *135*, 39–46. [CrossRef]
58. Kirunda, D.F.K.; McKEE, S.R. Relating quality characteristics of aged eggs and fresh eggs to vitelline membrane strenght as determined by a texture analyzer. *Poult. Sci.* **2000**, *79*, 1189–1193. [CrossRef]
59. Feddern, V.; De Prá, M.C.; Mores, R.; da Silveira Nicoloso, R.; Coldebella, A.; de Abreu, P.G. Egg quality assessment at different storage conditions, seasons and laying hen strains. *Ciência e Agrotecnologia* **2017**, *41*, 322–333. [CrossRef]
60. Al-Obaidi, F.A.; Shahrasad, M.J.; Al-Shadedi; Al-Dalawi, R.H. Quality, chemical and microbial characteristics of table eggs at retail stores in Baghdad. *Int. J. Poult. Sci.* **2011**, *10*, 381–385. [CrossRef]
61. Nadia, N.A.A.; Bushra, S.R.Z.; Layla, A.F.; Fira, M.A. Effect of coating materials (gelatin) and storage time on internal quality of chicken and quail eggs under refrigeration storage. *Egypt. Poult. Sci. J.* **2012**, *32*, 107–115.
62. Saleh, G.; El Darra, N.; Kharroubi, S.; Farran, M.T. Influence of storage conditions on quality and safety of eggs collected from Lebanese farms. *Food Control.* **2019**, *111*, 107058. [CrossRef]
63. Luo, W.; Xue, H.; Xiong, C.; Li, J.; Tu, Y.; Zhao, Y. Effects of temperature on quality of preserved eggs during storage. *Poult. Sci.* **2020**, *99*, 314–3157. [CrossRef] [PubMed]
64. Scott, T.A.; Silversides, F.G. The effect of storage and strain of hen on egg quality. *Poult. Sci.* **2000**, *79*, 1725–1729. [CrossRef]
65. Jin, Y.H.; Lee, K.T.; Han, Y.K. Effects of storage temperature and time on the quality of eggs from laying hens at peak production. *Asian-Aust. J. Anim. Sci.* **2011**, *24*, 279–284. [CrossRef]
66. Samli, H.E.; Agma, A.; Senkoylu, N. Effects of storage time and temperature on egg quality in old laying hens. *J. Appl. Poult. Res.* **2005**, *14*, 548–553. [CrossRef]
67. Coutts, J.A.; Wilson, G.C. *Optimum Egg Quality—A Practical Approach*, 1st ed.; 5M Publishing: Sheffield, UK, 2007; p. 64, ISBN 97-809-5301-506-1.
68. Eke, M.O.; Olaitan, N.I.; Ochefu, J.H. Effect of storage conditions on the quality attributes of shell (table) eggs. *Niger. Food J.* **2013**, *31*, 18–24. [CrossRef]
69. Santos, J.S.; Maciel, L.G.; Seixa, V.N.C.; Araújo, J.A. Parâmetros avaliativos da qualidade física de ovos de codornas (*Coturnix coturnix japonica*) em função das características de armazenamento. *Revista Desafios* **2016**, *3*, 54–67. [CrossRef]
70. Jones, D.R. Conserving and monitoring shell egg quality. In Proceedings of the 18th Annual Australian Poultry Science Symposium, Sydney, Australia, 20–22 February 2006; pp. 157–165.
71. Yimenu, S.M.; Koo, J.; Kim, J.-Y.; Kim, J.-H.; Kim, B.-S. Kinetic modeling impacts of relative humidity, storage temperature, and air flow velocity on various indices of hen egg freshness. *Poult. Sci.* **2018**, *97*, 4384–4391. [CrossRef] [PubMed]
72. Tyler, C.; Geake, F.H. The effect of water on egg shell strength including a study of the translucent areas of the shell. *British Poult. Sci.* **1964**, *5*, 277–284. [CrossRef]

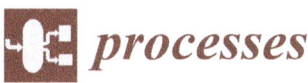

Article

Characterization of *Bacillus* Species from Market Foods in Beijing, China

Qiao Hu [1,2,†], Yuwen Fang [1,2,†], Jiajia Zhu [1,2], Wenjiao Xu [1,2] and Kui Zhu [1,2,*]

[1] College of Veterinary Medicine, China Agricultural University, Beijing 100193, China; huqiao@cau.edu.cn (Q.H.); fangyuwen@cau.edu.cn (Y.F.); zhujiajia@cau.edu.cn (J.Z.); xwjvet@163.com (W.X.)
[2] National Center for Veterinary Drug Safety Evaluation, College of Veterinary Medicine, China Agricultural University, Beijing 100193, China
* Correspondence: zhuk@cau.edu.cn
† These authors contributed equally to this article.

Abstract: Foodborne diseases have been witnessing a constant rising trend worldwide, mainly caused by pathogenic microorganisms, such as *Bacillus* spp., posing a direct threat to public health. The purpose of this study was to evaluate the biological risk of foodborne and probiotic *Bacillus* spp. in Beijing markets. A total of 55 *Bacillus* isolates, including 29 *B. cereus*, 9 *B. licheniformis* and 7 *B. subtilis*, mostly found in dairy products (32.7%), were recovered from 106 samples and identified by matrix-assisted laser desorption/ionization mass spectrometry and polymerase chain reaction methods. The susceptibility towards 16 antibiotics was determined using a broth microdilution method. *Bacillus* showed a high level of resistance to florfenicol (100%), lincomycin (100%), tiamulin (78.2%) and ampicillin (67.3%), while they were all susceptible or intermediate to vancomycin and rifampin. Additionally, we obtained the whole genome of 19 *Bacillus* strains using high-throughput sequencing, and the rates of resistance genes *van*, *fosB*, *erm* and *tet* were 57.9%, 57.9%, 21.1% and 26.3%, respectively. Moreover, 100%, 9.1%, 45.5% and 100% of these isolates carried virulence genes *nhe*, *hbl*, *cytK* and *entFM*, respectively. Lastly, 60% *Bacillus* strains were positive in hemolysis tests, and 3 *B. licheniformis* strains displayed an inhibitory activity on the growth of *S. aureus* ATCC 29213 using agar overlay technique. Our study outlines the characteristics of foodborne *Bacillus* spp. and provides information for the monitoring of food safety.

Keywords: emerging foodborne pathogens; *Bacillus*; probiotics; antimicrobial resistance

Citation: Hu, Q.; Fang, Y.; Zhu, J.; Xu, W.; Zhu, K. Characterization of *Bacillus* Species from Market Foods in Beijing, China. *Processes* **2021**, *9*, 866. https://doi.org/10.3390/pr9050866

Academic Editor: Nevijo Zdolec

Received: 15 April 2021
Accepted: 11 May 2021
Published: 14 May 2021

Publisher's Note: MDPI stays neutral with regard to jurisdictional claims in published maps and institutional affiliations.

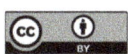

Copyright: © 2021 by the authors. Licensee MDPI, Basel, Switzerland. This article is an open access article distributed under the terms and conditions of the Creative Commons Attribution (CC BY) license (https://creativecommons.org/licenses/by/4.0/).

1. Introduction

Foodborne diseases are now a widespread and growing problem to public health and the world economy [1–3]. It is estimated that about 600 million people are suffering from foodborne illnesses, such as malaise, diarrhea, etc., which even stimulates the possibility of cancer, leading to 420,000 deaths annually [4,5]. Food safety hazards are associated with the ingestion of poisonous toxins, chemicals, and mostly bacteria, viruses, or parasites [6,7]. Notably, pathogens with the competence of producing toxins play a crucial role in foodborne illnesses [8].

Bacillus species are Gram-positive, spore-forming, rod-shaped, aerobic or facultative anaerobic bacteria, and they are ubiquitously distributed in soil, water, the environment as well as various food products [9,10]. By virtue of their multilayer-structured endospores, *Bacillus* spp. offer high tolerance towards acid, dehydration, γ-ray and ultraviolet radiation; they are stable during heat processing and low-temperature storage [11–14]. Several *Bacillus* strains have been screened for their potential probiotic functionalities in animal husbandry, bionematicides and antibiotic alternatives [15,16]. Additionally, they have also been verified to possess pathogen exclusion, anti-oxidant, immuno-modulatory and food fermentation abilities [17–20]. *Bacillus* and *Paenibacillus* spp. can yield potent antimicrobial lipopeptides, including polymyxins, octapeptins, polypeptins, iturins, surfactins, fengycins, tridecaptins and kurstakins, which are usually secondary metabolites produced by non-ribosomal peptide synthetases (NRPSs) [21]. A mixture of D- and L-amino acids equips those lipopeptides with an enhanced ability to withstand proteolytic enzymes from target organisms, as well as human plasma proteases, and potentially enables treatment by oral administration and intravenous injection [21–23].

Nevertheless, *Bacillus* is an opportunistic pathogen that may cause severe local or systemic infections, such as endophthalmitis and septicemia, when allowed access to mammalian tissues [16]. Few members of *Bacillus* spp., particularly *B. cereus* and *B. anthracis*, are infamous for producing emetic toxins (Cereulide) or enterotoxin. PA-LF (protective antigen- lethal factor) and PA-EF (edema factor) are *B. anthracis* generated toxins that induce the deadly disease anthrax in humans and animals [24,25]. Cereulide, produced by *B. cereus* and *B. weihenstephanensis*, is a major cause of foodborne intoxications through inhibiting the synthesis of RNA, causing expansion of mitochondria and formation of vacuoles in the protoplasm of target cells, thus bringing cell apoptosis and even fulminant liver failure [26,27]. Three enterotoxins of *B. cereus* that belong to the family of pore-forming toxins (PFTs), including non-hemolytic enterotoxin (Nhe), hemolysin BL (Hbl) and cytolysin K (CytK), are mainly responsible for diarrhea [28–30]. On the other hand, the presence of transferrable antimicrobial resistance genes (ARGs) will endow foods and probiotics containing *Bacillus* spp. as a reservoir for the transmission of antibiotic resistance [31,32]. Foodborne *Bacillus* spp. could serve as a vehicle to spread ARGs, while probiotic *Bacillus* spp. that are excreted through improperly treated animal waste would facilitate the horizontal gene transfer of mobile ARGs. Further, the emergence of antibiotic resistant strains, especially those resistant to multiple antibiotics, can cause routine treatments of *B. cereus* infection to fail [9,33,34]. Therefore, the mobile ARGs in *Bacillus* strains is another safety parameter that requires prompt attention.

The Centers for Disease Control and Prevention (CDC) website claimed that there were 619 confirmed *Bacillus*-related outbreaks from 1998 to 2015. *B. cereus* is also the second most frequently found causative agent of confirmed and suspected foodborne outbreaks (FBOs) in France after *Staphylococcus aureus* [35]. The European Union summary report on trends and sources of zoonoses, zoonotic agents and food-borne outbreaks reported a total of 287 outbreaks caused by *B. cereus* toxins involving 3073 cases (about 8% hospitalization) in European Member States (MSs) in 2014, whereas 291 outbreaks involving 3131 cases (with 3% hospitalization) were reported by nine MSs in 2015 [36]. It is elucidated that rice, pasta, pastry and noodles are associated with emesis, whereas vegetables, meat products and milk products are connected with diarrhea, based on previous epidemiological data [12,37]. Dairy products such as infant formula in the Chinese market have caused a considerable number of *B. cereus*-induced FBOs [38]. Furthermore, the diarrheal-type disease has been reported more frequently in Northern Europe, such as in Finland and Norway, as well as the emetic-type disease in Japan and the UK, constituting a great challenge both in developed and developing societies [39,40]. Our study aims to investigate the potential virulence, molecular characteristics and antibiotic resistance profiles of *Bacillus* spp. isolated from market foods in Beijing, China, providing information about the prevalence and pathogenicity of *Bacillus* spp. to further ensure food safety.

2. Materials and Methods

2.1. Sample Collection

From September to December in 2020, we collected a total of 106 samples, including 31 Beijing specialty food, 29 dairy products, 15 rice products, 11 probiotics, 9 fermented food, 7 raw or cooked meat, 2 soybean milk and 2 snacks from different local markets and restaurants in Beijing, China. All samples were independently kept in sealed, sterile plastic bags, transported directly to the laboratory within 24 h and stored at 4 °C or −20 °C.

2.2. Bacterial Isolation and Identification

Liquid samples were serial-decimally diluted as needed, and solid samples were suspended in phosphate-buffered saline (PBS, pH = 7.2) as initial dilution before being plated onto the surface of Brilliance *Bacillus cereus* Agar (Oxoid) and incubated at 37 °C for 24 h. Blue/green colonies were considered as presumptive *B. cereus*. The colonies were then transferred into 1 mL brain heart infusion (BHI, Land Bridge Technology) broth and incubated at 37 °C for 24 h (200 rpm). The bacterial cultures were spread on BHI agar, incubated at 37 °C for another 24 h, and single colonies were chosen for further study.

The species-specific identification was performed by ① matrix-assisted laser desorption ionization-time of flight mass spectrometry (AXIMA Performance, Shimadzu, Japan). First, bacterial samples were grown on BHA agar plates, and a single colony was selected and smeared directly as a thin film on the steel sample plate; 0.8 µL of 70% formic acid and 1 µL of CCA matrix solution (prepared with 50% acetonitrile and 2.5% trifluoroacetic acid in pure water) were then dropped onto the smear successively. The loaded sample plate was left for several minutes at room temperature to dry before inserting it into the AXIMA for data acquisition. ② 16S rRNA sequencing: From cultures grown overnight in BHI at 37 °C, DNA of each isolate was extracted by centrifuging at $5000 \times g$ for 5 min and resuspending in 50 µL Tris-EDTA (TE, Amresco) buffer. The suspensions were boiled in water bath at 100 °C for 10 min. Then. the tubes were placed on ice immediately for 10 min. The procedure was repeated twice, and samples were centrifuged at $14,000 \times g$ for 5 min to obtain the genomic DNA of each isolate. All the extracted DNA was stored at −20 °C; 16S rRNA sequence analysis was used to further characterize the *Bacillus*-like strains, using primers 27F and 1492R [41]. PCR products were sent to Tsingke Biological Technology (Beijing, China) for sequencing. Genomic sequences were identified in NCBI nucleotides databases using BLAST program (https://blast.ncbi.nlm.nih.gov/Blast.cgi). The strains with high similarity to 16S rRNA sequence of the reference strain (Evalue = 0 and Max identity ≥ 98%) were regarded as *Bacillus* spp. strains.

2.3. Antimicrobial Susceptibility Tests

The minimum inhibitory concentrations (MICs) of isolated *Bacillus* spp. towards 16 kinds of antimicrobial agents (ampicillin, ceftriaxone, gentamicin, streptomycin, kanamycin, erythromycin, tetracycline, florfenicol, ciprofloxacin, vancomycin, rifampicin, linezolid, lincomycin, tiamulin, chloramphenicol, amoxicillin + clavulanate) were tested using a standard broth microdilution method (Clinical and Laboratory Standards Institutes [CLSI] Supplement M100). *Staphylococcus aureus* ATCC 29213 was used as the quality control strain.

2.4. Genome Sequencing and Bioinformatics Analysis

Bacterial genomes of 19 *Bacillus* isolates were extracted using a bacterial genome DNA extraction kit (Tiangen Biotech, Beijing, China) and sequenced using the Illumina HiSeq ×10 system (Annoroad, Beijing, China). The draft assemblies of the sequences were obtained with SPAdes 3.0, and antimicrobial resistance genes and virulence genes were screened using Center for Genomic Epidemiology (CGE).

2.5. Hemolysis Test and Detection of Bacterially Produced Inhibitory Compounds

(a). The *Bacillus* strains were cultured on sheep blood agar plate (5%) to identify the hemolytic properties after incubation at 37 °C for 24 h.

(b). A single colony of *Bacillus* was inoculated into 1 mL of BHI broth. Incubation took place over night with shaking (200 rpm) at 37 °C; 5 µL of bacterial suspension was pipetted on the BHA plate, and it was dried in sterile air and incubated at 37 °C for 24 h. The upper MHA agar layer was seeded with *E. coli* ATCC 25922/*S. aureus* ATCC 29213, and it was incubated at 37 °C for 24 h after solidification. The production of antimicrobial agents was indicated by the inhibition zone.

3. Results

3.1. Sample Collection and Bacterial Composition

A total of 55 *Bacillus* isolates were obtained from 41 samples (38.7%), including 29 *B. cereus* strains, 9 *B. licheniformis* strains, 7 *B. subtilis* strains, 5 *B. pumilus* strains, 2 *B. amyloliquefaciens* strains, 1 *B. taeanensis*, 1 *B. velezensis* and 1 *Paenibacillus cookii* strain (Figure 1, Figure 2). Moreover, 18 isolates were recovered from dairy products, and 11 isolates were from local specialty foods (Table 1). We found that the dominant species was *B. cereus* in dairy products, rice products and Beijing specialty foods, while the proportion varied slightly from different sources. The major bacteria in fermented foods and probiotics were *B. pumilus* and *B. licheniformis*, respectively. Only 1 *B. subtilis* strain was isolated from a ham. No *B. cereus* strain was found in probiotic products (Figure 3). Detailed information about the food source of each strain is listed in Table S1 (Supplementary Material). Taken together, it is clarified that *Bacillus* spp. was a probable contaminant in market foods, and the main threat could be ascribed to *B. cereus*.

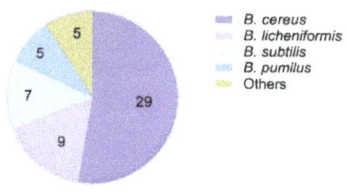

Figure 1. Proportion of different species of *Bacillus* isolates. *B. cereus*, *B. licheniformis*, *B. subtilis* and *B. pumilus* constitute 52.7%, 16.4%, 12.7% and 9.1% of the total number, respectively. Other species include *B. amyloliquefaciens* (3.6%), *B. taeanensis* (1.8%), *B. velezensis* (1.8%) and *Paenibacillus cookie* (1.8%).

Table 1. Number of samples and bacterial isolates of different sources.

Sample Source	No. of Samples	No. of Isolates
Beijing specialty food	31	11
Dairy products	29	18
Rice products	15	8
Probiotics	11	9
Fermented food	9	8
Raw or cooked meat	7	1
Soybean milk	2	0
Snacks	2	0
Total	106	55

Dairy products include pasteurized milk, yogurt and cheese; rice products include foods made from flour, rice, noodles and cakes; fermented foods include pickles, kimchi and preserved beancurd.

3.2. Antimicrobial Susceptibility of Bacillus Isolates

We subjected all the 55 isolates to antimicrobial susceptibility tests. Generally, *Bacillus* isolates showed complete resistance to florfenicol and lincomycin. The resistance rates towards ampicillin, amoxicillin + clavulanate and ceftriaxone were 67.3%, 54.5% and 70.9%, respectively (Figure 4). A large proportion of isolates exhibited resistance to streptomycin and tiamulin with levels of 56.4% and 78.2%. None of the isolates showed tolerance to either rifampin or vancomycin. It is noteworthy that all 29 *B. cereus* strains were resistant to ampicillin and ceftriaxone, while other *Bacillus* spp. were mostly sensitive to these two antibiotics (Table 2). *B. pumilus* isolates were susceptible to 12 antibiotics except for ceftriaxone, florfenicol, lincomycin and tiamulin. Compared with other *Bacillus* species, *B. cereus* showed more severe resistance to antibacterial agents. In terms of different food sources, *Bacillus* isolated from dairy products and rice products are highly resistant to penicillin–ampicillin and amoxicillin + clavulanate, for which isolates from vegetables, meat and probiotics displayed more sensitivity. *Bacillus* from probiotics expressed very low resistance to ampicillin, streptomycin, kanamycin, erythromycin, florfenicol, linezolid and lincomycin. Collectively, the presence of resistant strains revealed that antimicrobial resistance may have widely disseminated through *Bacillus* spp. in the food chain.

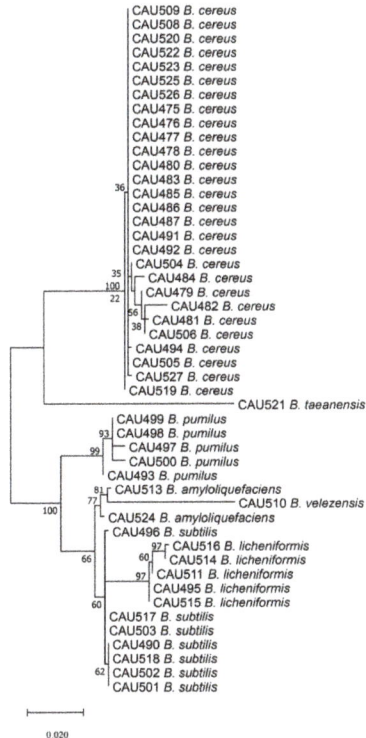

Figure 2. Phylogenetic tree of *Bacillus* isolates based on 16S rRNA sequences. The tree was constructed using maximum likelihood method, and genetic distances were generated using Kimura 2-parameter model. The numbers at the branches are bootstrap confidence percentages from 1000 bootstrapped trees.

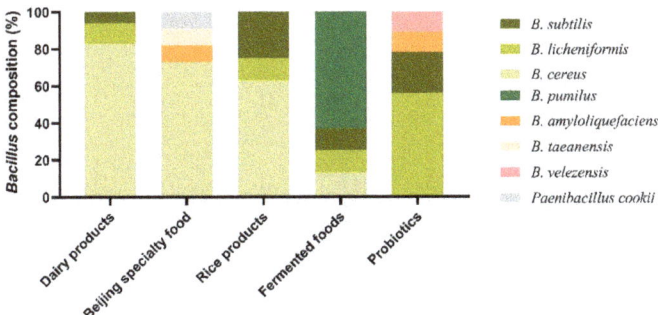

Figure 3. Compositions of *Bacillus* species in the samples from different sources. *B. cereus* is the dominant species in the isolates recovered from dairy products, Beijing specialty foods and rice products. *B. pumilus* and *B. licheniformis* are the most prevalent groups of fermented foods and probiotics-derived *Bacillus* strains, respectively.

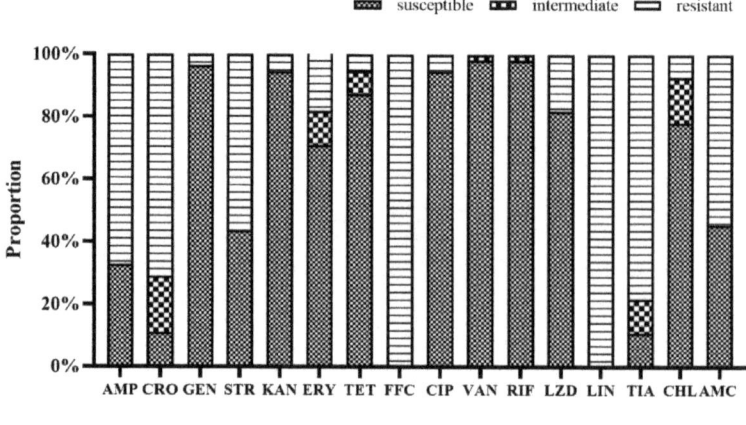

Figure 4. The proportions of susceptible, intermediate and resistant strains among 55 isolated *Bacillus* strains to 16 antibiotics. AMC: ampicillin, CRO: ceftriaxone, GEN: gentamicin, STR: streptomycin, KAN: kanamycin, ERY: erythromycin, TET: tetracycline, FFC: florfenicol, CIP: ciprofloxacin, VAN: vancomycin, RIF: rifampicin, LZD: linezolid, LIN: lincomycin, TIA: tiamulin, CHL: chloramphenicol, AMC: amoxicillin + clavulanate.

Table 2. Proportion of *Bacillus* strains of different species resistant to antibiotics.

Antibiotics	Fraction of Resistant Isolates			
	B. cereus	*B. licheniformis*	*B. subtilis*	*B. pumilus*
AMP	29/29	3/9	1/7	0
CRO	29/29	3/9	1/7	5/5
GEN	2/29	0	0	0
STR	15/29	7/9	7/7	0
KAN	1/29	1/9	0	0
ERY	2/29	7/9	0	0
TET	2/29	0	0	0
FFC	29/29	9/9	7/7	5/5
CIP	2/29	0	0	0
VAN	0	0	0	0
RIP	0	0	0	0
LZD	6/29	1/9	3/7	0
LIN	29/29	9/9	7/7	5/5
TIA	23/29	9/9	4/7	4/5
CHL	1/29	2/9	0	0
AMC	29/29	0	0	0

3.3. The Antimicrobial Resistance and Virulence Genes of Bacillus Isolates

According to the results of MIC tests, 19 *Bacillus* isolates were subjected to next-generation sequencing, and the whole genomic sequences were screened for ARGs and virulence genes. It is interpreted that 57.9%, 26.3% and 21.5% of *Bacillus* strains carried fosfomycin resistance gene *fosB*, tetracycline resistance gene *tet* and erythromycin resistance gene *erm*, respectively (Table 3). Vancomycin resistance gene *van* was present in 11 (100%) *B. cereus* isolates. In addition, 2 *B. subtilis* strains and 1 *B. pumilus* strain were found to harbor kanamycin resistance gene *aadK*, and 1 *B. pumilus* isolated from fermented vegetable and 1 *B. cereus* from dairy product carried chloramphenicol resistance gene *cat*. There was a poor consistency between the phenotypical and genetic antimicrobial resistance traits of tested strains. Interestingly, *B. cereus* was the only species carrying virulence genes, with the rates of 100%, 9.1%, 45.5% and 100% for *nhe*, *hbl*, *cytK* and *entFM*, respectively. Other virulence factor related genes include *PLC*, *hlyIII*, *clo*, *InhA2*, and so on. Therefore, *Bacillus* spp. derived from foods are likely to develop resistance to drugs and produce toxins that cause relevant disease.

Table 3. The antibiotic resistance genes and virulence genes of *Bacillus* isolates.

Strains	Species	Sources	ARGs	VGs
CAU475	B. cereus	Dairy products	fosB, van	clo, entFM, hlyIII, inhA2, nheA, nheB, nheC, nprA, PLC, sph
CAU476	B. cereus	Dairy products	fosB, tetA, van	clo, cytK, entFM, entS, hlyIII, inhA2, nheA, nheB, nheC, nprA, PLC, sph
CAU479	B. cereus	Dairy products	fosB, van	clo, cytK, entFM, entS, hlyIII, inhA2, nheA, nheB, nheC, nprA, PLC, sph
CAU480	B. cereus	Dairy products	aac, cat, fosB, van	clo, entFM, entS, hlyIII, inhA2, nheA, nheB, nheC, nprA, PLC, sph
CAU481	B. cereus	Dairy products	fosB, van	clo, cytK, entFM, entS, hlyIII, inhA2, nheA, nheB, nheC, nprA, PLC, sph
CAU482	B. cereus	Dairy products	fosB, van	clo, entFM, entS, hlyIII, inhA2, nheA, nheB, nheC, nprA, PLC, sph
CAU484	B. cereus	Dairy products	fosB, van	cesH, entFM, entS, hlyIII, inhA2, nheA, nheB, nheC, nprA, PLC, sph
CAU486	B. cereus	Dairy products	fosB, van	cesH, entFM, entS, hlyIII, inhA2, nheA, nheB, nheC, nprA, PLC, sph
CAU504	B. cereus	Rice products	fosB, van	clo, entFM, entS, hblA, hblC, hblD, hlbB, hlyIII, inhA2, nheA, nheB, nheC, nprA, PLC, sph
CAU505	B. cereus	Rice products	fosB, van	clo, cytK, entFM, entS, hlyIII, inhA2, nheA, nheB, nheC, nprA, PLC, sph
CAU506	B. cereus	Rice products	fosB, tetL, van	clo, cytK, entFM, entS, hlyIII, inhA2, nheA, nheB, nheC, nprA, PLC, sph
CAU495	B. licheniformis	Fermented vegetable	ermD	–
CAU511	B. licheniformis	Probiotics	ermD	–
CAU514	B. licheniformis	Probiotics	ermD	–
CAU516	B. licheniformis	Probiotics	ermD	–
CAU498	B. pumilus	Fermented vegetable	aadK, mphK, tetL	–
CAU500	B. pumilus	Fermented vegetable	cat	–
CAU501	B. subtilis	Ham	aadK, mphK, tetL	–
CAU502	B. subtilis	Rice products	aadK, mphK, tetL	–

ARGs = antimicrobial resistance genes; VGs = virulence genes.

3.4. The Hemolytic Ability and Antibacterial Effect of Bacillus Isolates

Cytotoxicity is an important factor involved in pathogenesis of bacterium. We found that 33 out of the 55 (60%) *Bacillus* strains caused hemolysis. Among the hemolytic isolates, 75.8% were *B. cereus*, which was recognized as a dangerous pathogen correlated with food poisoning. All 5 *B. pumilus* strains were hemolytic, while *B. licheniformis* were completely non-hemolytic. Of seven *B. subtilis* strains, two resulted in hemolysis, suggesting that a large number of *Bacillus* spp. have the capability of rupturing red blood cells.

We observed that 3 *B. licheniformis* strains (CAU495, CAU511, CAU514) exerted an inhibitory effect on the growth of *S. aureus* ATCC 29213, and none of the bacteria inhibited *E. coli* ATCC 25922 (Figure 5). *B. licheniformis* CAU495, CAU511 and CAU514 were obtained from fermented vegetables, pet probiotics and livestock probiotics, respectively, with diameters of the zone presented to be 2, 1.1 and 1.9 cm. Thus, foodborne *Bacillus* spp. showed the potential of developing into a probiotic strain.

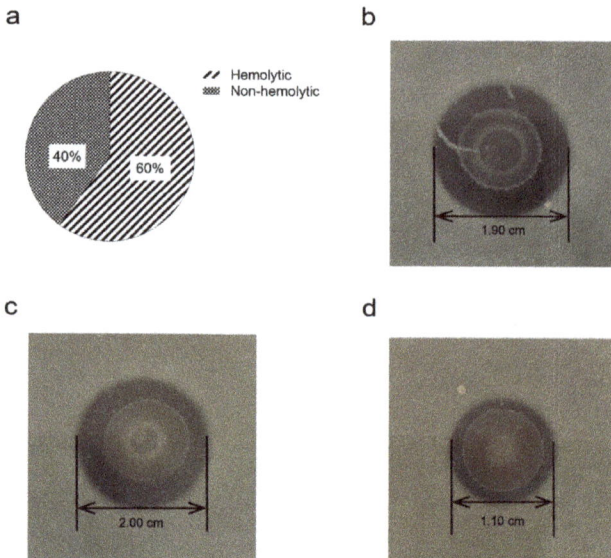

Figure 5. Results of the hemolysis test and agar overlay technique. (**a**) proportion of hemolytic and non-hemolytic *Bacillus* strains; 60% of *Bacillus* strains were hemolytic on sheep blood. (**b–d**) are the inhibition zones of *B. licheniformis* CAU514, CAU495 and CAU511, respectively, with *S. aureus* ATCC 29213 added in the soft-agar overlay.

4. Discussion

Our study confirmed the presence of *Bacillus* spp. in several kinds of foods. The highest prevalence was in dairy and rice products, illustrated by the antimicrobial resistance of 55 *Bacillus* isolates mainly towards florfenicol, lincomycin and florfenicol and lincomycin. Meanwhile, the virulence genes were common in *B. cereus*, and 3 out of 55 strains displayed the capability of attacking other organisms. In spite of the rapid advancement in the fields of food science and technology, and a growing concern raised by various international groups on food safety, prevalence of foodborne illness still remains a substantial cause of morbidity and preventable mortality [42]. *Bacillus* is designated as a group of soil inhabitants that also can be isolated from varied sources including vegetables and food. It represents the most heterogeneous group considering their phenotypic and genotypic characters. Some distinct species such as *B. cereus* have also been recognized as opportunistic pathogens or toxin producers in human or animal hosts. In this study, we collected 95 food samples from local markets in Beijing and 11 probiotic products purchased from other areas. A total of 55 *Bacillus* strains were obtained from 41 samples, mostly composed of *B. cereus* (29/55). Among different categories of food products, dairy products were the most important niche, followed by specialty foods, probiotics and rice products. However, Beijing specialty foods are theoretically a sub-type of rice products, which implies that both rice products and dairy products were eligible residences for *Bacillus* spp. In Japan, *B. cereus* was found in 66 out of 101 (65.3%) domestically pasteurized milk samples, which is moderately higher than the rate (51.7%) of our study [43]. In addition, a previous study found that nearly half of the 65 isolated *Bacillus* spp. strains from 34 commercial probiotic products harbored multiple antimicrobial resistance genes, coupled with mobile genetic elements, and were capable of producing hazardous toxins, while no *B. cereus* was recovered from the 11 probiotics we collected, indicating that those samples were free from the contamination of *B. cereus* and its toxins [44].

We found that 55 *Bacillus* isolates were all resistant to florfenicol, lincomycin and had significant resistance to tiamulin, ampicillin, amoxicillin + clavulanate and ceftriaxone.

Since *B. cereus* are able to produce β-lactamase, they are intrinsically resistant to β-lactams. It is also reported that ABC (ATP binding cassette) efflux transporters of *B. subtilis* can generate tolerance to lincosamide, which is consistent with our results [45]. Concerning the resistance genes, we disclosed that *B. cereus*, *B. subtilis* and *B. licheniformis* mainly carried fosfomycin resistance gene *fosB*, tetracycline resistance gene *tet* and erythromycin resistance gene *erm*, separately. *B. cereus* isolates, obtained from vegetables in South Korea, were susceptible to imipenem, vancomycin, gentamicin, erythromycin, ciprofloxacin and chloramphenicol, and unlike the tendency of our results, 40.5% from romaine lettuce were resistant to rifampin and 6% of isolates from garlic chives exhibited resistance to tetracycline [46]. Moreover, 147 *B. cereus* sensu lato strains isolated from German market food showed resistance against the β-lactam antibiotics such as penicillin G and cefotaxim (100%), as well as amoxicillin/clavulanic acid combination and ampicillin (99.3%), while most strains were susceptible to ciprofloxacin (99.3%), chloramphenicol (98.6%), imipenem (93.9%), erythromycin (91.8%), gentamicin (88.4%) and tetracycline (76.2%), which are higher than our results to a mild extent [47]. Our findings suggest that *Bacillus* is a group of potential foodborne pathogens harboring mobile ARGs and might undermine the therapeutic effect of antibiotics.

B. cereus produces a wide array of virulence factors, including pore-forming toxins, cereulide, hemolysins, enterotoxins, proteases and phospholipases [48]. We discovered here that virulence genes were undetectable in *Bacillus* spp., except *B. cereus*. The detection rates of *nhe*, *hbl* and *cytK* were 100%, 9.1% and 45.5%, respectively, and *ces* was 0. Another study focusing on *B. cereus* in Chinese markets, distinguished by the sample volume (860) and sites (39 cities), revealed that 35% of ready-to-eat (RTE) food was contaminated with *B. cereus*, with 39%, 83%, 68% and 7% of the isolated strains harboring the enterotoxin-encoding gene clusters *hblACD*, *nheABC*, *cytK* and emetic toxin-encoding gene *cesB*, respectively. The majority of the isolates were resistant to most β-lactam antibiotics and rifamycin [49], which is largely consistent with our findings. From 2013 to 2015, Kui Zhu et al. isolated 18 *B. cereus group* strains from 15 probiotics and discovered that all strains produced the enterotoxin Nhe, 15 strains additionally produced Hbl, and nearly half of them harbored the antimicrobial resistance gene *tet(45)* [50]. In Egypt, 6.9 and 8.5% of *B. cereus* were recovered from milk powder and Ras-cheese, respectively, and *nhe* gene was detected and dominated in all isolates (100%) from both products [51]. A South Korean survey involving 496 samples of food from environmental and clinical origin, found that 92.3% and 59.5% of *B. cereus* strains carried *nhe* and *hbl*, respectively [52]. Those studies have presented that almost all *B. cereus* harbor the *nhe* gene, including the emetic *B. cereus*, which explains that vomiting symptoms are often accompanied with diarrhea. Regarding the hemolytic activity, most *B. cereus* could destroy blood cells, denoting their virulence towards target cells to some extent. Apart from the biological perils that have been discussed, we found encouraging evidence of 3 *B. licheniformis* strains that showed antimicrobial activities towards Gram-positive bacteria, indicating the potential of being probiotic candidates or antibiotic alternatives. Thus, among isolated *Bacillus* strains, *B. cereus* constitutes a principal part in generating antimicrobial resistance and virulence. Other species of *Bacillus* spp., on the other hand, have different phenotypical features and could even release antibacterial components.

5. Conclusions

Our findings connote that *Bacillus* spp. are distributed in a variety of food products with a potential of secreting virulent substances and disseminating antimicrobial resistance. They are also possible resources for new antibiotic substitutes. Therefore, corresponding guidelines regarding the sterilization, pasteurization and monitoring of toxins in the whole food chain, especially on-shelf foods, should be developed to further promote public health.

Supplementary Materials: The following are available online at https://www.mdpi.com/article/10.3390/pr9050866/s1, Table S1: Food sources of each *Bacillus* strain.

Author Contributions: Conceptualization, Q.H. and Y.F.; methodology, Q.H.; software, Q.H.; validation, Q.H. and Y.F.; formal analysis, Q.H. and J.Z.; investigation, Q.H. and Y.F.; resources, W.X.; data curation, Q.H. and Y.F.; writing—original draft preparation, Q.H. and Y.F.; writing—review and editing, W.X. and J.Z.; visualization, J.Z.; supervision, K.Z.; project administration, K.Z.; funding acquisition, K.Z. All authors have read and agreed to the published version of the manuscript.

Funding: This research was funded by the National Key Research and Development Program of China (2017YFC1600305), Beijing Municipal Science and Technology Project (Z201100008920001) and Beijing Dairy Industry Innovation Team.

Institutional Review Board Statement: Not applicable.

Informed Consent Statement: Not applicable.

Conflicts of Interest: The authors declare no conflict of interest.

References

1. Bennett, S.D.; Sodha, S.V.; Ayers, T.L.; Lynch, M.F.; Gould, L.H.; Tauxe, R.V. Produce-associated foodborne disease outbreaks, USA, 1998–2013. *Epidemiol. Infect.* **2018**, *146*, 1397–1406. [CrossRef]
2. Schlinkmann, K.M.; Razum, O.; Werber, D. Characteristics of foodborne outbreaks in which use of analytical epidemiological studies contributed to identification of suspected vehicles, European Union, 2007 to 2011. *Epidemiol. Infect.* **2017**, *145*, 1231–1238. [CrossRef]
3. Li, W.; Pires, S.M.; Liu, Z.; Ma, X.; Liang, J.; Jiang, Y.; Chen, J.; Liang, J.; Wang, S.; Wang, L.; et al. Surveillance of foodborne disease outbreaks in China, 2003–2017. *Food Control* **2020**, *118*, 107359. [CrossRef]
4. World Health Organization. Food Safety. Available online: https://www.who.int/news-room/fact-sheets/detail/food-safety (accessed on 30 April 2020).
5. Mughini-Gras, L.; Schaapveld, M.; Kramers, J.; Mooij, S.; Neefjes-Borst, E.A.; Van Pelt, W.; Neefjes, J. Increased colon cancer risk after severe *Salmonella* infection. *PLoS ONE* **2018**, *13*, e0189721. [CrossRef] [PubMed]
6. Cao, Y.; Feng, T.; Xu, J.; Xue, C. Recent advances of molecularly imprinted polymer-based sensors in the detection of food safety hazard factors. *Biosens. Bioelectron.* **2019**, *141*, 111447. [CrossRef] [PubMed]
7. Fung, F.; Wang, H.-S.; Menon, S. Food safety in the 21st century. *Biomed. J.* **2018**, *41*, 88–95. [CrossRef]
8. Rajkovic, A.; Jovanovic, J.; Monteiro, S.; Decleer, M.; Andjelkovic, M.; Foubert, A.; Beloglazova, N.; Tsilla, V.; Sas, B.; Madder, A.; et al. Detection of toxins involved in foodborne diseases caused by Gram-positive bacteria. *Compr. Rev. Food Sci. Food Saf.* **2020**, *19*, 1605–1657. [CrossRef] [PubMed]
9. Bottone, E.J. *Bacillus cereus*, a Volatile Human Pathogen. *Clin. Microbiol. Rev.* **2010**, *23*, 382–398. [CrossRef]
10. Nicholson, W.L. Roles of *Bacillus* endospores in the environment. *Cell. Mol. Life Sci.* **2002**, *59*, 410–416. [CrossRef]
11. Drobniewski, F.A. *Bacillus cereus* and related species. *Clin. Microbiol. Rev.* **1993**, *6*, 324–338. [CrossRef]
12. Kotiranta, A.; Lounatmaa, K.; Haapasalo, M. Epidemiology and pathogenesis of *Bacillus cereus* infections. *Microbes Infect.* **2000**, *2*, 189–198. [CrossRef]
13. Vidic, J.; Chaix, C.; Manzano, M.; Heyndrickx, M. Food Sensing: Detection of *Bacillus cereus* Spores in Dairy Products. *Biosensors* **2020**, *10*, 15. [CrossRef] [PubMed]
14. Nicholson, W.L.; Munakata, N.; Horneck, G.; Melosh, H.J.; Setlow, P. Resistance of *Bacillus* endospores to extreme terrestrial and extraterrestrial environments. *Microbiol. Mol. Biol. Rev.* **2000**, *64*, 548–572. [CrossRef] [PubMed]
15. Bader, J.; Albin, A.; Stahl, U. Spore-forming bacteria and their utilisation as probiotics. *Benef. Microbes* **2012**, *3*, 67–75. [CrossRef] [PubMed]
16. Elshaghabee, F.M.F.; Rokana, N.; Gulhane, R.D.; Sharma, C.; Panwar, H. *Bacillus* as potential probiotics: Status, concerns, and future perspectives. *Front. Microbiol.* **2017**, *8*, 1490. [CrossRef] [PubMed]
17. Lefevre, M.; Racedo, S.M.; Ripert, G.; Housez, B.; Cazaubiel, M.; Maudet, C.; Jüsten, P.; Marteau, P.; Urdaci, M.C. Probiotic strain *Bacillus subtilis* CU1 stimulates immune system of elderly during common infectious disease period: A randomized, double-blind placebo-controlled study. *Immun. Ageing* **2015**, *12*, 1–11. [CrossRef]
18. Shobharani, P.; Padmaja, R.J.; Halami, P.M. Diversity in the antibacterial potential of probiotic cultures *Bacillus licheniformis* MCC2514 and *Bacillus licheniformis* MCC2512. *Res. Microbiol.* **2015**, *166*, 546–554. [CrossRef] [PubMed]
19. Ripert, G.; Racedo, S.M.; Elie, A.-M.; Jacquot, C.; Bressollier, P.; Urdaci, M.C. Secreted Compounds of the Probiotic *Bacillus clausii* strain O/C inhibit the cytotoxic effects induced by *Clostridium difficile* and *Bacillus cereus* toxins. *Antimicrob. Agents Chemother.* **2016**, *60*, 3445–3454. [CrossRef]
20. Terlabie, N.N.; Sakyi-Dawson, E.; Amoa-Awua, W.K. The comparative ability of four isolates of *Bacillus subtilis* to ferment soybeans into dawadawa. *Int. J. Food Microbiol.* **2006**, *106*, 145–152. [CrossRef]
21. Cochrane, S.A.; Vederas, J.C. Lipopeptides from *Bacillus* and *Paenibacillus* spp.: A gold mine of antibiotic candidates. *Med. Res. Rev.* **2016**, *36*, 4–31. [CrossRef]
22. Zhao, H.; Shao, D.; Jiang, C.; Shi, J.; Li, Q.; Huang, Q.; Rajoka, M.S.R.; Yang, H.; Jin, M. Biological activity of lipopeptides from *Bacillus*. *Appl. Microbiol. Biotechnol.* **2017**, *101*, 5951–5960. [CrossRef] [PubMed]

23. Bareia, T.; Pollak, S.; Eldar, A. Self-sensing in *Bacillus subtilis* quorum-sensing systems. *Nat. Microbiol.* **2018**, *3*, 83–89. [CrossRef] [PubMed]
24. Jennings-Antipov, L.D.; Song, L.; Collier, R.J. Interactions of anthrax lethal factor with protective antigen defined by site-directed spin labeling. *Proc. Natl. Acad. Sci. USA* **2011**, *108*, 1868–1873. [CrossRef] [PubMed]
25. Toh, M.; Moffitt, M.C.; Henrichsen, L.; Raftery, M.; Barrow, K.; Cox, J.M.; Marquis, C.P.; Neilan, B.A. Cereulide, the emetic toxin of *Bacillus cereus*, is putatively a product of nonribosomal peptide synthesis. *J. Appl. Microbiol.* **2004**, *97*, 992–1000. [CrossRef] [PubMed]
26. Andersson, M.A.; Hakulinen, P.; Honkalampi-Hämäläinen, U.; Hoornstra, D.; Lhuguenot, J.-C.; Mäki-Paakkanen, J.; Savolainen, M.; Severin, I.; Stammati, A.-L.; Turco, L.; et al. Toxicological profile of cereulide, the *Bacillus cereus* emetic toxin, in functional assays with human, animal and bacterial cells. *Toxicon* **2007**, *49*, 351–367. [CrossRef] [PubMed]
27. Rouzeau-Szynalski, K.; Stollewerk, K.; Messelhäusser, U.; Ehling-Schulz, M. Why be serious about emetic *Bacillus cereus*: Cereulide production and industrial challenges. *Food Microbiol.* **2020**, *85*, 103279. [CrossRef] [PubMed]
28. Tran, S.-L.; Guillemet, E.; Ngo-Camus, M.; Clybouw, C.; Puhar, A.; Moris, A.; Gohar, M.; Lereclus, D.; Ramarao, N. Haemolysin II is a *Bacillus cereus* virulence factor that induces apoptosis of macrophages. *Cell. Microbiol.* **2010**, *13*, 92–108. [CrossRef] [PubMed]
29. Jeßberger, N.; Dietrich, R.; Bock, S.; Didier, A.; Märtlbauer, E. *Bacillus cereus* enterotoxins act as major virulence factors and exhibit distinct cytotoxicity to different human cell lines. *Toxicon* **2014**, *77*, 49–57. [CrossRef]
30. Dietrich, R.; Jessberger, N.; Ehling-Schulz, M.; Märtlbauer, E.; Granum, P.E. The food poisoning toxins of *Bacillus cereus*. *Toxins* **2021**, *13*, 98. [CrossRef]
31. Berendonk, T.U.; Manaia, C.M.; Merlin, C.; Fatta-Kassinos, D.; Cytryn, E.; Walsh, F.; Buergmann, H.; Sørum, H.; Norström, M.; Pons, M.-N.; et al. Tackling antibiotic resistance: The environmental framework. *Nat. Rev. Microbiol.* **2015**, *13*, 310–317. [CrossRef] [PubMed]
32. Cabello, F.C.; Godfrey, H.P.; Buschmann, A.H.; Dölz, H.J. Aquaculture as yet another environmental gateway to the development and globalisation of antimicrobial resistance. *Lancet Infect. Dis.* **2016**, *16*, e127–e133. [CrossRef]
33. Friedman, N.; Temkin, E.; Carmeli, Y. The negative impact of antibiotic resistance. *Clin. Microbiol. Infect.* **2016**, *22*, 416–422. [CrossRef]
34. Nolte, O. Antimicrobial resistance in the 21st century: A multifaceted challenge. *Protein Pept. Lett.* **2014**, *21*, 330–335. [CrossRef] [PubMed]
35. Glasset, B.; Herbin, S.; Guillier, L.; Cadel-Six, S.; Vignaud, M.-L.; Grout, J.; Pairaud, S.; Michel, V.; Hennekinne, J.-A.; Rama-Rao, N.; et al. *Bacillus cereus*-induced food-borne outbreaks in France, 2007 to 2014: Epidemiology and genetic characterisation. *Eurosurveillance* **2016**, *21*. [CrossRef] [PubMed]
36. European Food Safety Authority; European Centre for Disease Prevention and Control. The European Union summary report on trends and sources of zoonoses, zoonotic agents and food-borne outbreaks in 2016. *EFSA J.* **2017**, *15*, e05077. [CrossRef]
37. Anderson Borge, G.I.; Skeie, M.; Sørhaug, T.; Langsrud, T.; Granum, P.E. Growth and toxin profiles of *Bacillus cereus* isolated from different food sources. *Int. J. Food Microbiol.* **2001**, *69*, 237–246. [CrossRef]
38. Liu, X.-Y.; Hu, Q.; Xu, F.; Ding, S.-Y.; Zhu, K. Characterization of *Bacillus cereus* in dairy products in China. *Toxins* **2020**, *12*, 454. [CrossRef]
39. Jessberger, N.; Dietrich, R.; Granum, P.E.; Märtlbauer, E. The *Bacillus cereus* food infection as multifactorial process. *Toxins* **2020**, *12*, 701. [CrossRef] [PubMed]
40. Bennett, S.D.; Walsh, K.A.; Gould, L.H. Foodborne disease outbreaks caused by *Bacillus cereus*, *Clostridium perfringens*, and *Staphylococcus aureus*–United States, 1998-2008. *Clin. Infect. Dis.* **2013**, *57*, 425–433. [CrossRef] [PubMed]
41. Lane, D.J. *16S/23S rRNA Sequencing. Nucleic Acid Techniques in Bacterial Systematic*; Wiley: Chichester, UK; New York, NY, USA, 1991; pp. 115–175.
42. Akhtar, S.; Sarker, M.R.; Hossain, A. Microbiological food safety: A dilemma of developing societies. *Crit. Rev. Microbiol.* **2012**, *40*, 348–359. [CrossRef]
43. Shimojima, Y.; Kodo, Y.; Soeda, K.; Koike, H.; Kanda, M.; Hayashi, H.; Nishino, Y.; Fukui, R.; Kuroda, S.; Hirai, A.; et al. Prevalence of Cereulide-producing *Bacillus cereus* in pasteurized milk. *Shokuhin Eiseigaku Zasshi* **2020**, *61*, 178–182. [CrossRef] [PubMed]
44. Cui, Y.; Wang, S.; Ding, C.; Shen, J.; Zhu, K. Toxins and mobile antimicrobial resistance genes in *Bacillus* probiotics constitute a potential risk for One Health. *J. Hazard. Mater.* **2020**, *382*, 121266. [CrossRef] [PubMed]
45. Ohki, R.; Tateno, K.; Takizawa, T.; Aiso, T.; Murata, M. Transcriptional termination control of a novel ABC transporter gene involved in antibiotic resistance in *Bacillus subtilis*. *J. Bacteriol.* **2005**, *187*, 5946–5954. [CrossRef]
46. Park, K.M.; Jeong, M.; Park, K.J.; Koo, M. Prevalence, enterotoxin genes, and antibiotic resistance of *Bacillus cereus* Isolated from raw vegetables in Korea. *J. Food Prot.* **2018**, *81*, 1590–1597. [CrossRef]
47. Fiedler, G.; Schneider, C.; Igbinosa, E.O.; Kabisch, J.; Brinks, E.; Becker, B.; Stoll, D.A.; Cho, G.-S.; Huch, M.; Franz, C.M.A.P. Antibiotics resistance and toxin profiles of *Bacillus cereus*-group isolates from fresh vegetables from German retail markets. *BMC Microbiol.* **2019**, *19*, 250. [CrossRef] [PubMed]
48. Enosi Tuipulotu, D.; Mathur, A.; Ngo, C.; Man, S.M. *Bacillus cereus*: Epidemiology, virulence factors, and host–pathogen interactions. *Trends Microbiol.* **2021**, *29*, 458–471. [CrossRef]
49. Yu, S.; Yu, P.; Wang, J.; Li, C.; Guo, H.; Liu, C.; Kong, L.; Yu, L.; Wu, S.; Lei, T.; et al. A Study on prevalence and characterization of *Bacillus cereus* in Ready-to-Eat foods in China. *Front. Microbiol.* **2020**, *10*, 3043. [CrossRef] [PubMed]

50. Zhu, K.; Hölzel, C.S.; Cui, Y.; Mayer, R.; Wang, Y.; Dietrich, R.; Didier, A.; Bassitta, R.; Märtlbauer, E.; Ding, S. Probiotic *Bacillus cereus* strains, a potential risk for public health in China. *Front. Microbiol.* **2016**, *7*, 718. [CrossRef]
51. Abdeen, E.E.-S.; Hussien, H.; Hadad, G.A.E.; Mousa, W.S. Prevalence of virulence determinants among *Bacillus cereus* isolated from milk products with potential public health concern. *Pak. J. Biol. Sci.* **2020**, *23*, 206–212. [CrossRef] [PubMed]
52. Forghani, F.; Kim, J.-B.; Oh, D.-H. Enterotoxigenic profiling of emetic toxin- and enterotoxin-producing *Bacillus cereus*, isolated from food, environmental, and clinical samples by multiplex PCR. *J. Food Sci.* **2014**, *79*, M2288–M2293. [CrossRef]

MDPI
St. Alban-Anlage 66
4052 Basel
Switzerland
Tel. +41 61 683 77 34
Fax +41 61 302 89 18
www.mdpi.com

Processes Editorial Office
E-mail: processes@mdpi.com
www.mdpi.com/journal/processes

www.ingramcontent.com/pod-product-compliance
Lightning Source LLC
LaVergne TN
LVHW070601100526
838202LV00012B/531